ESCAPING
the *FOG*

ESCAPING *the* FOG

by
Shawn Beddingfield

Published by Best Seller Publishing®, Pasadena, CA
Best Seller Publishing® is a registered trademark
Printed in the United States of America.
ISBN 9798667949343

For more information, please write:
Best Seller Publishing®
253 N. San Gabriel Blvd, Unit B
Pasadena, CA 91107
or call 1(626) 765 9750
Visit us online at: www.BestSellerPublishing.org

Contents

Preface

This book is structured in the format of a 12-step-meeting "share." *What it was like, what happened, and what it's like now.* A share can be when a person is invited to speak at a meeting for around 20 minutes compared to the three-to-five-minute share given during the open discussion part of a meeting. The author has chosen to open up and speak honestly and show vulnerability out of a desire to help others see the similarities that the disease of alcoholism displays in most of those who suffer from the affliction. More importantly, if you happen to struggle with alcoholism, this sharing is to empower you, the reader, to arrive at the determination that you are not in this fight alone.

Alcoholism is a common affliction, and there are some people who have been able to discover a solution. The 12-step program has proven successful for those individuals who can be honest with themselves. Fighting this disease has been shown to have greater success when the sufferer involves him- or herself with a group of people who are familiar with the disease and have found success staying sober themselves by working with other addicts.

As is true for most addicts, the author started his journey into oblivion looking to mask trauma—in his case, the death of his baby sister. Numbing comfort from the pain is what alcohol and drugs provided for the author, and everything seemed good, until it just wasn't. This led to a lifelong battle with substance abuse, culminating in his finally achieving sobriety.

The last part of this book discusses the redemption of self-worth the author experienced in the form of training for and completing a series of five triathlons over six months during the spring and summer of 2019. Training and competing in endurance sports helped focus his nervous energy on something positive, and he came to understand that kicking an addiction takes action—life-habit-changing action. If you are struggling with addiction, you are not alone.

What it was like, what happened, and what it's like now.

I was sitting on the edge of the bed trying to muster up a good cry, but I just couldn't find the tears. It was late September of 2016. I had just been brought into the detox room reserved for new clients at the rehab in Napa. I couldn't help laughing at the irony of rehabbing in California's wine region. When the staff member who showed me to my room just behind the kitchen asked me if I needed anything, I responded with, "a towel please," because I knew I was going to cry.

I wasn't sure why; it just seemed like the appropriate thing to do. Was it because I was going to be away from my wife and kids for the next 30 days? That would be, by far, the longest we were ever apart. Or was it because my relationship with alcohol, my lifelong mate, was about to come to an end? (This still wouldn't be the end of my drinking, but my current sobriety would start within six months.)

I asked myself how I got here. Was it the lost loves of the past? Was it my divorce from G.? Was it the irregular heartbeat that led to my minor stroke just two years prior? Was it the near-death experiences? Most recently, the hemoglobin level of 5, which was well below the healthy level 11, that required immediate blood transfusion to stave off death? Was it the stroke at age 49? Or was the alcohol just not working for me anymore? They say it's all good until it's not.

All I knew was I just couldn't live the way I had been any longer. I was on the verge of my second divorce. My children had lost all respect for me. My oldest, 13 at the time, wrote me a letter describing how she was too afraid to bring friends over to the house after school out of fear that I would already be drunk. She told me how embarrassed she was of me and that if I didn't do something, she would. I took that to mean she would harm herself or run away.

I had previously purchased a prepaid cremation plan on monthly installments and was afraid I would die before it was paid off. I wasn't sure how my wife was going to get the insurance money before I needed to be cremated. I figured she would have to figure it out. I didn't think I was going to be there to walk my girls down the aisle at their weddings, and the way things were going, I might not even be invited to do so if I were still alive.

In the years prior, I had tried rehab three times through the facilities covered by my insurance. I enrolled in two three-day-a-week outpatient programs and one two-week, all-day outpatient program in Oakland. I had to get up at 5:30 to catch the 6:30 BART train in order to be on time in Oakland. Driving home from the BART station, I found my car seemed to be preprogrammed to make a hard-right turn into the am/pm where I used to buy beer on my way home from the BART train returning from Oakland. On more than one occasion, I stopped in, but I got only a six pack.

In Oakland, they Breathalyzed and piss-tested us randomly. I flunked three tests. They offered to send me to an inpatient rehab years earlier, but it was the holidays, and I still wasn't done. When I was finally ready for rehab I had recently sold a home and was going to use the commission to pay for a trip to Disneyland during the fall break in October. I would end up having to use the Disneyland money to pay for rehab. My family was disappointed but decided they would rather have a sober daddy than spend another week with a drunk daddy in Disneyland.

If you're anything like me, at times you may feel that there is no hope, that you're not worthy of any better. I am not going to tell you if I can get sober, then you can too. I am not sure what your circumstances are. I can say with confidence, though, that because of my experience, I know it can be done. I didn't think I had a hope in hell. My life was beyond repair. But with the help of God and a 12-step program, I was able to achieve about three years of sobriety.

When I first got sober, I didn't think I was ever going to have fun again. Life as I knew it was over. At the time, that thought had negative implications. But now, I live a life of freedom beyond my wildest dreams. My family adores me, and we laugh and love most all the time. It's not perfect. What is? But it's better than it was. I no longer miss alcohol; I no longer have cravings. That's not to say that occasionally I don't have what I call *memory cravings*; like on New Year's Day, after taking all the Christmas boxes to the recycle center and mowing the lawn, I felt like it was time for college football and a cold beer. But that thought passed quickly, and I felt much better afterward. This book would still be stuck in my brain's fog if I weren't sober.

They have speaker meetings at the 12-step group I attended. We were asked to explain *what it was like, what happened, and what it's like now*. So that is the format of this book, they call it a share; this book is a share. They also encourage you to share your courage, strength, and hope, and I hope you'll find that in the following pages. Most of all, understand that I didn't start out wanting to be part of that fellowship. I wasn't one of "those" guys. It wasn't until I was completely willing to embrace the program and become one of those guys that I was finally able to get sober. Those guys became my friends, my support, and without them, I wouldn't be where I am today.

Later in the book, I'll get to *what happened*. Let me just say, though, that I couldn't get sober until I admitted to myself that I am different; I cannot drink like a normal person. Racing from point A to point B, totally stressed, hands shaking with the anticipation of a drink, and then the need to drink more, to get drunker, drink faster—my mind was completely obsessed.

Writing this book was not easy. I'm not looking for sympathy, but I had to go back into deep, dark places to retrieve memories that would have been best left in the past. I did it because I thought it would be helpful to myself, and perhaps, somebody else who may see their own actions in my past. The final step of the program, the 12th step, encourages participants to give back to those who still suffer.

For most, that means working as a *sponsor* to help a newcomer travel through the 12 steps. Working together can help both parties stay sober. For me, I want to encourage you to participate, if you feel you may need help. The only requirement for membership to this fellowship is a *desire* to quit drinking. If you have a desire, you belong.

The fellowship is anonymous, so they don't advertise. But you can find them close to the front of the phone book. If you can't seem to find the help, don't hesitate to reach out to me. I will gladly help put you in contact with your local fellowship.

CHAPTER 1
In the Beginning —Life at Home

Some of my greatest mentors have said "start with the end in mind." So as I sit down to write this book, I see the end of the process as you reading it. I was born on May 5, 1965, in Fremont, California. My older sister, Tracey, was a year old, and my mother and father had moved out from the East. My biological dad, who I didn't meet until I was about 13, lived in Warrenville, Illinois. I saw him only twice in my life, at 13 and 14, and since I had already started spiraling out of control, that relationship never blossomed. He told me we would never be friends, that he would always be my dad and only a dad. Since up to that point, all I knew was he was a shit-dad, that didn't pan out as a beneficial relationship for either of us.

My grandparents that I never met owned a bowling alley with a bar, and my grandpa was a local politician in the community, I have been told. Thinking about my lineage—*politician, bar owner*—those sound like vocations instilled in my genes. It's kind of ironic that a bar is where I would have some of my best times and some of my worst, and I always fancied myself a would-be politician. I became a bartender in my 20s. It seems appropriate now. In retrospect, it's almost like I was genetically predetermined to follow this family path.

My mother grew up in Pennsylvania and met my dad when she was in beauty college in Philadelphia. He was on weekend leave with the Navy. I don't know all the gory details, but let's just say my sister Tracey and I were a catalyst and result of their union. They ended up in Naperville, Illinois, and for reasons I'm not aware of, moved to the Bay area after the birth of my sister but before my birth.

Apparently, my dad was very popular in Warrenville and knew most of the people in town. When my parents moved West, my father discovered that he was no longer the "mayor" of the town and wanted to move back to Illinois. But my mom was quite content to stay in California where she had family. After leaving a note for my mother outlining his intentions, my father headed to the airport with me and Tracey in tow to fly home.

She didn't want any part of that scenario, so she sent my Uncle Dick to the airport to cut him off. I never met or saw my dad again until I was about 13 years old. After that, I spent a total of about three weeks with him; he died when I was 35. I attended his funeral, which had a military honor guard, as well as a police escort since he was a police officer. He was also a volunteer firefighter. I learned more about his character from the eulogies at his funeral than I had ever known.

My mother stayed in California and met Bob, who became my second father from ages two to six. He was my hero as well. I remember admiring him for being a great water-skier who even built his own boat. Athletics and camping were passions we both shared. One of my first memories was of Bob dangling me over the edge of the boat into the cold, deep, dark-blue Lake Shasta. It was so terrifying that I'm amazed I ended up being the water lover I am.

I was able to get very good at water-skiing, just like Bob. It was always one of my favorite things to do, and I did it most everywhere I went. Bob and my mom separated and divorced when I was about six. When my Mom took me kicking and screaming from the house, I was so upset I threw up all over the front seat of her car. I was devastated. If the death of my younger sister was the switch that triggered my addictive personality, then being taken from the person who, as far as

I was concerned, was "my father" was the back-up switch that could have activated my addiction. Having life as you know it end abruptly can kind of distract one's focus.

I saw Bob only a couple of times after that, when I was in in my mid-teens, and then, one time after that when I was in my 20s at my house in San Jose. He ended up owning a gym. Again, ironic that, although I was not from his gene pool, it would have seemed appropriate for me to have inherited those genes.

During this time in my life, I had a babysitter I knew as Auntie Liz (no relation, just the babysitter). She had an older son who raced quarter midgets. Auntie Liz and her husband, "Uncle Don," were a big part my life at that time. Don tried to plop me down behind the wheel of a quarter midget cart one day, and I cried like a baby and refused to drive. And it's really too bad because I believe I could have been a great race-car driver and probably would have ended up preceding Jeff Gordon as the best driver from the Greater Bay Area.

It turned out my mom left Bob to be with stepdad #2, Jim Beddingfield, who ended up being my stepdad from ages 6 until about 14. Jim was the manager of a local chain store (W.T. Grants or something like that). We ended up in an apartment in San Jose after a couple of nights in motels. The early honeymoon period with Jim was all ice cream and puppies. But that soon gave way to "the conversation," in which Jim informed Tracey and me that if we did not heed his warnings, "that's one strike." On the third strike, we were subject to three spankings. This became a routine that regularly struck the fear of God in me, but didn't seem to dissuade Tracey or me from our overall behavior. Now would be a good time to point out that Tracey and I never really got along and were constantly fighting.

I do remember a time when I was playing at a neighborhood friend's house and I got into a fight with my sister. I don't recall what the fight was even about, but I remember the imminent spanking. Jim counted me out and told me to go home and "get ready" for a spanking. I was so scared I went home and put on a dozen pairs of underwear, thinking I'd finally found a way to outsmart him. When Jim got home,

I got my first whack. No response. Then, no response to the second whack. When the third whack failed to rattle me, he figured something was up. He grabbed the waistbands of the underwear by the handful, and before I could say a thing, I was "bare-ass" and getting a licking I would not soon forget.

At seven, I joined a swim team and practiced swimming at the house of a fellow named Coach Bell. After a year or two, I found myself winning most of the races I entered and enjoying myself in the process. This lasted the better part of my young competitive swimming career. It was about then that I started noticing girls. With my tan swimmer's body and sun-faded blonde hair, they noticed me too. I was a gregarious kid who loved the spotlight of winning.

I remember two times when the whole team was let out of practice early because I was able to achieve a goal set by the coach. The first was to swim the 50-yard pool, underwater without air. The second was to do seven push-up dips on the railing of the pool stairs. Both times I accomplished the goal to a resounding response from the team. My swimming career peaked at about age nine or ten, when two of the hot 15-year-old girls greeted me at the end of the final race of the year and declared me champion. It was in *breaststroke*, which was not lost on my prepubescent mind.

However, in the start of the next season, my grip on first place began to slip. In that second summer, day-practice took off at five in the morning. I was so cold in the pool that my only warmth stemmed from the tears streaming down my cheeks. My desire to compete was starting to diminish, and the results followed. A couple of years later, my mom asked me if I still wanted to swim. Not knowing if she was just pulling my leg, I responded with a resounding "heck no."

At first, giving up being the "mayor" of the swim team was a hard adjustment to make. By then, my half-sister, Heather, was born. Heather was the bright spot in the brutal environment that Jim had created. She had curly, red hair and blue eyes. I took her on walks and pretended her stroller was a 4x4 truck. She also had fair skin, and her lips and fingernail beds were blue. She was soon diagnosed with having a hole in her heart that needed to be surgically repaired. It was supposed to be a routine surgery, performed by one of the best surgeons in the field at the time. But on July 7, 1977, my life took a terribly tragic turn. Shortly after Heather's surgery, she was rushed back into the operating room, where she internally bled out and choked on her own blood.

For years, I would be chasing the brief joy I knew before her death. It was around this time in my life that I realized I had an abundance of energy and was very fidgety in school, and that I got my first taste of beer. I was at a family wedding and a guy named BoBo gave me half of a can of Coors beer. I can remember driving home from Fremont to San Jose sitting in the backseat of Jim's car just feeling completely relaxed—no sadness, stress, or anxiety from the drive; everything was peaceful. It wouldn't be too much longer before the addiction to drugs and alcohol would have me in its grips.

Before that happened, I struggled in school. It started with my being kept out of most of my eighth-grade school year with a platelet disorder that manifested with symptoms of leukemia. I was put on large doses of steroids, and the puffiness and weight-gain associated with those medications soon started. I started to fall behind and never really caught up.

My self-image as that tan, toned stud of a kid was replaced by that of a chunky, pale introvert. It didn't help that Jim and my mom moved us from the Blossom Valley of San Jose, a blue-collar neighborhood, to the Almaden Valley, better known as the "Golden Ghetto." BMWs and kegger parties were the norm at my new school.

At 14, I realized that, as a new kid, I could choose my own image—*cool kid* was it. While ninth grade had its challenges, the fact that I was determined to be cool helped. At the time, I was a Raider fan, and the quarterback Kenny Stabler was my hero. Rumor had it that Kenny would party Saturday nights in Tahoe and still win games on Sunday. That was when I decided I was going to show people you didn't need to be a jock to succeed at sports. Being able to party your ass off and still perform was way cooler. I would spend the better part of my athletic life trying to prove this theory. My other hero at the time was Burt

Reynolds. *Smokey and the Bandit* was a hit movie. Drink. Drive. Get the girl. My kind of guy.

School was becoming more and more challenging, and my interests in the social aspects of school rather than the curriculum didn't help. Back then, ADD (attention deficit disorder) was not a well-known diagnosis. Turns out that a combination of everything I had been through and good old genetics made me a poster boy for the disorder. All those years spent swimming probably blunted the head of that spear, but once I quit swimming, that energy built.

I remember being called into the vice principal's office in tenth grade and asked if I had any idea why I was testing second-year, college-level comprehension in English on the State assessment test but flunking my English class. I had an idea but just couldn't put my finger on it.

I wanted to play on the football team and went out to the bleachers for the tryout meeting, but lost my courage and ended up slithering away halfway through the meeting. Football was my favorite sport at the time, and I regret not hanging in there. At this point in my life, I understand that if I had played football, I may not be writing a book about my endurance sports endeavors because I could have blown out my knees at some point during my football career. I guess I'll never know.

Of course, by then I had started partying on the weekends at keg parties and smoking pot. I either drank or smoked. Never both. I was too smart. At that point, my drinking went from 0 to 100, lickety-split. Drunk was never drunk enough, and puking was a constant thing. I started smoking pot in the morning (wake and bake), midday, and evenings. Did I leave anything out? I had the standard addict thought "I can quit anytime, just not now."

In tenth grade, I was dating a cheerleader, which fulfilled my orchestrated image. Junior year, I played the field and joined the track team. I ran the 400 and practiced with the cross-country team. That was my first taste of distance running. I never made it to a meet because my desire to stop midway through a distance run and get stoned overpowered my desire to compete.

By senior year, I had the first "love of my life." Julie was a junior and the youngest of three sisters. She was the only one left at home by then, so her parents were lax about her coming and going. We spent many nights together. At that point, my mom and Jim were divorced, and she was sowing her own wild oats. I was living a 17-year-old boy's dream. Although I went to school most every day, I did not always make it to class, and inevitably, I did not graduate. I finished my high school days as a member of the FFA Club which in my case stood for Future F*#k Up of America. When I was voted both Class Clown and Biggest Flirt, the yearbook advisor anointed me "Most Unforgettable."

I may not have amounted to much academically, but the social aspect of school that I chose to fulfill was a success. That and a buck purchased me plenty of coffees after that. My mom was the best friend a guy could have. I always had a car or truck and had everything I needed; maybe not wanted, but needed.

I started working at a gas station in high school with my sister's drug-salesman boyfriend. Then I moved up to a job at an upscale restaurant in a local hotel. I wore a dinner jacket and learned the finer points of fine dining. I always had tip money to supply my habit, and most of the people I worked with partied as well. I would leave the restaurant by the airport and drive, stoned out of my mind, past the police station home to Almaden, where Julie often waited up for me.

In the winter following high school, I decided to move to Lake Tahoe. I have always loved Tahoe, and that's where I wanted to live. Even though I'd had rough times with Mom, moving out of the house was one of the toughest decisions I ever made. It was four hours away, and Tracey was on the verge of moving out also. That's not the last time I would ever live with Mom, but it was a big change at the time.

I moved to my Uncle Dick's cabin. He was the one who almost kicked my dad's ass for trying to take me back to Illinois as a baby. Julie had decided to move to Wisconsin to live with her sister, relegating us to long-distance status, and since *long distance* was not unlimited back then, this became very expensive very fast. My Uncle Dick should probably have kicked me out the first time he got a $200-plus bill.

The movie, *Ski Patrol*, had come out, depicting mountain-life as *wine, women, and song* (and Jacuzzis). Julie broke up with me, and soon thereafter, I adopted it as theme of life. Since Mom wasn't going to foot the bill, I needed a job. Heavenly Valley was hiring. I took their aptitude test and was called into a conference room with nine other people. The HR representative explained there were four jobs on the California side and four jobs on the Nevada side. I scored sixth, so I was looking at a job as a chairlift operator on the Nevada side, which might as well have been Siberia.

The first four candidates took the California side, as expected. The HR representative then turned to me, paused, and said, "You know, we do have a job on the Tram. Would you be interested in that, Shawn?"

The Tram, at the time, was the showcase of the mountain on the California side, and I pounced on that opportunity. Once again, everything changed. From the Tram, I was able to meet most of the "cool" local skiers. My life rapidly evolved from Bay area transplant to local. It would have been quite different otherwise. For better or for worse, I guess I'll never know.

CHAPTER 2

Life on the Mountain

After spending my first winter on the Tram at Heavenly, hobnobbing with the locals and improving my skiing, I decided to stay on at Heavenly for the summer season. The Tram closed for a couple of months while the snow was melting, so I went to work with the trail crew. We put in the perimeter for Mott Canyon, a triple black diamond ski run on the Nevada side of the mountain.

After being flown by helicopter to the top, we took drops of twenty-foot-long poles in bundles of six. We would take a drop and work our way in treacherous terrain 120 feet to the next drop. Then we were flown by helicopter from the bottom of the canyon back to the top, where we worked our way back down the canyon, spacing the poles out every twenty feet.

We spent the next couple of days playing mountain goat, lugging a posthole auger and digging holes in the mountain. After we were done, it was time to go back to the Tram for summer duty. On summer Tram duty, we shuttled people from the parking lot to the top of the Tram restaurant. On the way down, I would play "Sailing" by Christopher Cross, hypnotizing the riders with the combination of the song and the view. I timed the song so that the piano end was synchronized with the

Tram car as it slowed and rocked into its stall. By the end of the season, I must have heard that song hundreds of times.

That summer, I spent much of my alone-time with Veronica, the second "love of my life," also known as *the one that got away*. I met Veronica during the winter, but it wasn't until the summer that she started riding the Tram with me, more often than was necessary. I was so ignorant and intimidated by her blonde hair and green eyes that I assumed she was just riding the Tram out of boredom. I became good friends with Vern, who later dubbed me "shy Shawn" to her friends. This was very much the beginning, and far from the end, of our story.

Toward the end of the summer, a friend of mine, who was also named Shawn, came to visit. We went to Angora Lakes for the day to jump off the cliffs, about a 60-foot drop. We were doing our thing when a girl came to my attention. As soon as I saw her, I told Shawn, "That is the girl I am going to marry."

Katie was visiting from Michigan. She and her friend Lisa were staying at a cabin at the lake. I struck up a conversation with the girls and convinced them to come have dinner with us at the cabin. The only thing I remember about that night was the fact that the chicken from the grill was raw (I have since mastered BBQ) and that Katie ended up spending the night with me. Just a couple of months later, Katie packed up and moved from Michigan to live with me in Tahoe, thus becoming "Love of My Life #3."

I was still living at my Uncle Dick's cabin in Meyers, or should I say below the cabin. My place could best be described as a studio on the *basement* level of the cabin. When I say basement, it was not like an East Coast converted basement but more like living under the main cabin floor, where the cabin was built on stilts to conform with the grade of the mountain. It had enough room for a bed, a small bathroom with a stall shower, and a sink with a small stove.

At one point during the summer, before Katie moved in, Uncle Dick let the propane go empty, and I took cold showers for twenty days straight. Let me tell you, Tahoe water is butt-arse cold. Maybe that was Uncle Dick's way of telling me it was time to go. It wasn't long after Katie moved in that she read a diary I had from when I was a kid. Apparently, the night that Reggie Jackson hit three home runs in a World Series game ('77), I was drunk. Combining that with intimate knowledge of my daily activities, Katie was the first person who ever accused me of being an alcoholic. While I was aware at that point that I probably had a problem, I still believed I could quit at any time. I just didn't want to! How dare she challenge that.

In my second winter in Tahoe, I continued working at Heavenly but switched from Tram to snowmaking. By then, Katie and I had moved to the bottom of "Killer" Keller Ave on Pioneer Trail with Tony, a guy I had worked with during my summer on the Tram. Keller had a 15–25 percent grade leading into the back entrance to Heavenly Valley. I had finally made it to Tahoe proper. Tony was a small-time pot dealer so there was a constant supply of the ganja.

My first year doing snowmaking was brutal. We worked from seven at night until seven in the morning, five days a week. The only good thing was that I was able to ski for a couple of hours most days, elevating my skiing skills to expert level. I don't believe I am any more talented than the next guy, but if you were to ski as much as I did, you would be pretty darn good too. The other great thing about snowmaking was "gun check." We checked the guns throughout the night in teams of two. Since most of the other guys smoked pot too, we would stop off at chairlift shacks or in the woods to get baked. We also got to ride snowmobiles, which allowed me to see some of the most beautiful sunrises over Nevada from 10,000 feet.

My first year, I was just a grunt with a dick supervisor who would walk by and kick your chair if you started to doze off. I would become supervisor in my second year and changed that. That winter, I also worked with Bruce, who lived across the street from the one-bedroom on Alameda Street where Katie and I ended up moving, closer to the lake. We called him the "Bruce of Abuse," and his roommates, C Rat (Chris) and Schmelly (Chris). They had all moved up from the Bay area a few years earlier and were considered locals at that point. The house they lived in was affectionately known as the Rat Pad.

By now, my relationship with Katie was deteriorating. Most of my time was spent at the Rat Pad getting drunk and stoned, working, or skiing on the slopes. I was also seeing a lot of Veronica. As I mentioned earlier, that story wasn't over. Needless to say, Katie was rapidly growing tired of my act, and I wasn't sure whether I wanted to be tied down to her. So much for getting married, which was what Katie wanted. She also wanted me to be sober. Katie and I had a healthy, intimate relationship when it was just us, but the combination of my working nights and her working days and my trips to the Rat Pad put a stress on our relationship. That and my immaturity and unwillingness to settle down.

One weekend, some high school friends came up to visit. In order to hold my honor as the life of the party, I was going to be the one to show them the town. They picked me up to go to the Casino. After a spat with Katie over my going out, I left her with some choice words and took the keys to our only vehicle (my truck) for good measure. We started the night drinking beer and getting stoned. Then, I proceeded to sit at the blackjack table and drink about 15 brandy separators. I will never know what possessed me to drink those. I never did before or since.

By six in the morning, there were only a couple of my friends still out. Forgetting I had told Katie off hours earlier, I called and asked her to come get us, to which she replied, "You took the keys, Dumbass." My friends and I started off walking down by the lake. There were patches of snow and it was pretty darn cold, and we had no jackets. At one point in our trek, we had to walk around a chain-link fence jutting out into the lake about knee-deep. I believe there was also a strand of barbed wire involved, since I still have a scar that looks like a mosquito bite on my leg I received from a poke.

After about a mile and a half of the four-mile journey, we wandered out to Highway 50, realizing that, while the lake was beautiful, it was not the best route. I stopped at the nearest pay phone (remember those?) and called Katie and apologized profusely. I begged her to come rescue us. This would not be the last time that I would call someone I had pissed off in my drunken stupor and ask her to come rescue me.

About twenty minutes later, and not too much closer to home, a cab passed going the other way. The cab made a U-turn, and pulled up next to us on the curb. It was Katie. She came. *I still got it.* Returning home, we sent my friends off in the cab. I returned the keys to Katie, and she went off to work, while I passed out on the couch.

Sometime during my slumber (I was on my back), I felt a warm, slimy sensation in my throat. Not enough to wake me, but I was aware. I started to choke and finally rolled over on my side. I was on the verge of dying like the rock star I thought I was, by choking on my own puke. When Katie got home, she discovered me still passed out. I had projectile-vomited all over the front room, walls, and television. Everywhere. Believe it or not, Katie forgave me, and we stayed together.

My second summer in Tahoe, I decided I would be better off working at the lake, so I got a job at the marina. This time, I was hired as a "dock monkey," in charge of checking people in and out of their rented boats. But fate took over. On my second day, the longtime mechanic, Don (lost one eye in a Mexican prison, no time for that story), lost his black Lab and left the marina, quite pissed off, without her. As luck would have it, about 20 minutes later, the dog showed up, and I held her while Doug, the marina manager, called Don. Don came racing into the parking lot, skidded to a stop, got out of his truck, grabbed the dog by the collar and threw her into the front of the truck; he then drove off without saying a word to me.

The next day, Doug called me into the office and told me that Don requested an assistant and I was it. Once again, my life changed in an instant. I'm sure the job as dock monkey would have been fun but monotonous. Instead, I had a great summer, riding the rental Jet Skis and waterskiing and windsurfing.

Vern stopped by, every now and then, and Don would tell me to go "test a boat" and take her with me. Again, I thought she was just bored, never considering that she was probably into me. I was still too intimidated by her beauty to find out. I was still trying to stay loyal to

Katie, although by then, we were more roommates than lovers. At one point, Don told me I needed to quit playing house and either marry her or move out. I decided I just wasn't ready to commit to marrying Katie, so I broke up with her and moved across the street to live on the couch at the Rat Pad.

For my third winter in Tahoe, I decided to make a change and work at one of Don's friend's ski shop. I had moved to a room at a house across the street from the lake, which was essentially a tool shed in the backyard. I had to walk across the backyard to the house to go to the bathroom. Sometimes I just opened the door of the shed and relieved myself into the backyard.

It just so happened that my neighbor was one of the biggest coke dealers in town and my roommate and him were best buds. Things were out of control. I can remember being so hungover, one morning, that I went behind the skis hanging from the ceiling, grabbed a garbage can, and started puking my brains out. The owner of the shop came from the front of the store and shook his head at me with a look of disgust on his face. That was the end of that job.

By now, it was halfway through the winter, so I went back to snowmaking. Since the weather was getting warmer (above 30 degrees), it was like having a part-time job. I spent more time skiing than working. Between the winter and the summer, I started working at the local liquor store. It was like being a kid in a candy shop. I used to frequent a club on the Nevada side that was called the "After Dark" because we partied the nights away and walked out into morning. I was still playing the field and not making safe choices in my interactions with women. Katie was still in Tahoe, but we never saw each other. The closest I got to be around her was the night her roommate (who had the hots for me) made me dinner.

Around the holidays, one of my best friends from high school and his former coke-dealing boss came up to visit. Between him and my neighbor, it was a "white" Christmas. I had started dating a girl who was in an episode of "CHiPs" when she was younger. Dumb as a brick but hot as hell. One day, the coke dealer was missing an "eight-ball" or an eighth ounce of coke he had left in the bathroom drawer. Around the same time, the girl I was dating became impossible to find. The last time I saw her was when I went to reclaim the thousand-dollar chain I had bought her on credit for Christmas, and she looked pretty coked out.

After that, my friend who had moved from San Jose to Long Beach insisted that I go with him to Long Beach to straighten out my life. He encouraged me to enroll at Long Beach City College with him. I obliged with what was to be my first of many geographical moves, in which the intention was to get clean and sober.

My friend lived with another friend from high school in an apartment building owned by his dad. I enrolled in LBCC and started working with him and his dad at the ownership group. I did screens on buildings throughout Long Beach, Orange County, and the Inland Empire. It was not too long after my arrival that I hooked up with another high school friend who always had herb and a good connection. So much for getting clean.

I found out from another friend who had visited Katie in Tahoe that she was pregnant. I was devastated. The messed-up, delusional person I was thought we were living in a soap opera and we would eventually get back together. Since I was so immature at that point, a kid was a deal-breaker, and a heartbreaker.

Soon after, my friend introduced me to crack. As much of an addict as I was, it didn't take me long to realize *that shit* was just plain wrong. Thank God, that was a very short-lived phase. Long Beach was fun. I waterskied in the marina and went to school, but after a prolonged drought with the ladies, I decided to do another geographic move back to San Jose at the end of the semester.

As I mentioned, leaving home to move to Tahoe did not mark the last time I would live with my mom. At this point, I moved back home. My mom lived in an apartment, stumbling distance from the Britannia Arms on Almaden Expressway, which was a hangout for all my high school partier friends. I started bartending at a brand-new Chevy's Mexican Restaurant just down the street. Again, I was a kid in a candy store. This defeated my most recent attempt to get sober. I had made friends with the Red Lobster bartender at the restaurant across the parking lot and had already been friends with the guys at the "Brit." In the bartender culture, reciprocation and comps were seen as an honored professional courtesy. Same old story—wine, women and song.

Katie had moved back to Michigan and had a baby boy; she named him Shane. I can't tell you how many times I went through the math in my head to determine if there were any way Shane could have been mine. It just wasn't in the math.

During the summer, I dated a couple of girls, but nothing escalated to the level of couple. Then, after a summer of heavy drinking and smoking, I decided to move back to Tahoe. I was accepted back as a snowmaker based on my experience. This was going to be it; I was going to focus on work and skiing. I stayed back at the Rat Pad for a few weeks but then found a studio apartment in the Tahoe Keys with a view of Mt. Tallac. There was a boat dock and indoor pool down the street and tennis courts across the street. Other than swimming occasionally in the indoor pool, it was hard to keep up the illusion that I was still an athlete. It was fall, and boating season was over; I didn't even own a tennis racket.

By the end of the first month at Heavenly, I was promoted to co-supervisor with Jake. It came with the honored "Supervisor's Spider Jacket." It was navy blue with diagonal red stripes on the sleeves. This was seen as a status symbol. Getting baked in the chairlift shacks was still par for the course and worth a king's ransom from the other workers. Drinking was not only tolerated by the locals, but we were even viewed as local heroes. To show their appreciation, they often bought us post-shift beers to get us through the morning drought. The Bruce of Abuse had gone to work with C-Rat at the ski shop down the street from the Rat Pad.

After a mild winter, I got in plenty of skiing and was well entrenched with the locals as a "Face Rat." Because the black diamond run above the parking lot, the "Gunbarrel," was also referred to as

"The Face," we were known as "Face Rats." By the end of that winter, I had started skiing in the weekly Wednesday competition called the "Battle on the Barrel."

Since work was predicated upon freezing temperatures at night, we knew when the temperature was warm, we wouldn't have to work the next day. I would get my twenty dollars' worth of Heavenly Bucks from HR, which got me pitchers of beer for 50 percent off. There was beer and live music, and of course, plenty of tourist ski bunnies (wine, women, and song).

I hooked up with a girl who had a son the same age as Shane. On nights when we worked, I went down the mountain to visit her during my break, after her son went to bed. This was a very casual arrangement and never elevated to couple status. I had been back in touch with Katie, in the meantime, and there was talk of reconciliation. She decided to come out from Michigan to visit, and we would see how things went.

On the day she arrived, I made the mistake of lending my truck for the day to the girl I was having the fling with. When Katie arrived by cab, she immediately asked where my truck was. I had no explanation. Soon after, my truck and its driver showed up. The women saw each other at the door, and I was between a rock and a hard spot, unable to explain the situation away. I never saw Katie after that. We spoke a dozen times, but that ship had sailed. Since the affair was on unofficial terms, she didn't mind. That arrangement continued on for a bit longer.

After a few months of part-time working due to warm weather, my beer-and-weed budget was running trim. I solved that problem by moving out of my $800/month apartment in the Keys and selling the truck my mom had bought me during my last year of high school to my landlord. By this point, I was too good to drink and drive, so I just quit driving, leaving me plenty of cash to enjoy summer. Since the Bruce of Abuse had moved back to the Bay area, I was able to get my own room at the Rat Pad for the first time. I went back to work for the off-season at the liquor store, and it was back to more of the same.

In my third summer, I went to work for Dave, the owner of the Jet Ski rental company at the marina. This was awesome. Most days consisted of waking up around seven, going waterskiing on Schmelly's boat with him and C Rat. Some days, I was too hungover to put on my wet suit and I would just ski naked. I may have ski-streaked past the Edgewood Golf course at one point, and no, I never got water up my arse. From there, I would go and teach windsurfing from 9 to 12.

When hungover, which was most days, I dreaded the first 45 minutes of the lesson, spent on the shore on the simulator. The rest of the lesson, I could lie on a board and float, just using my arms. After work, I rode the Jet Ski for half an hour to an hour. By the end of summer, I was pretty good. Of course, I got baked throughout the day. After Jet Skiing, I rode my bike around South Shore and visited friends (and Vern). By then, the wind would be coming up, and I would go windsurfing for a couple of hours. Spending all that time on the water, I got pretty good at windsurfing.

Most days, after windsurfing, I'd grab another 30 minutes on the Jet Ski. The biggest decision I had to make every day was what I was having for dinner and who I was going to have it with. After dinner, C Rat would give me a few bong rips to do the dishes, and we all settled in for the night, drinking beer and watching an HBO movie. After the movie, we'd watch the news and then head off to our rooms to wake up at seven the next day and repeat the cycle.

This was pretty much how the summer went. I had a couple of dates and perhaps a couple of make-out sessions, but certainly never a girlfriend. And of course, none of this was with Veronica.

CHAPTER 3

Moving South

I was on the verge of what would be my final year in Tahoe. For the winter, I went back to snowmaking, still as a supervisor. The biggest change was this year we would be able to ski the face at night. We would use miner's lights, and the lowest part of the mountain was lit. I was still living at the Rat Pad, and since I had sold my truck, I was now relegated to riding my bike to work. Since I was busy drinking and smoking pot, driving, and for that matter, dating, was not a high priority. During the day going skiing, I could take the free Heavenly shuttle that picked up every half hour on the corner.

One of the worst parts of my mornings was at about six o'clock, when they would start the buses in the lower lot and the diesel smoke would drift uphill to where my crew and I would be watching the resort come alive. On an empty stomach, I would get nauseated by the fumes. As I mentioned earlier about not being a dick supervisor, I had implemented a policy where the crew took turns getting 30–60 minutes of sleep during their "lunch break" most nights. This wasn't necessarily endorsed by management, but it just seemed right at the time (and labor laws being what they are now, in retrospect).

This went a long way toward keeping the crew fresh, and it was much better than being startled awake if you happened to dose off, like that dick supervisor would do to me. It was also at that time that

I implemented another rule that was not endorsed by management. One of the worst tasks was at the end of the night when we would have to roll up thousands of feet of fire hose we used with the guns. I would tell the guys that if they were done by the time I went to the Top of the Tram restaurant and filled a five-gallon water jug half full of beer and returned, we would go to the top of the mountain, 10,000 feet, get baked, and watch the sun rise over Nevada. They never failed to finish the task.

I used to tell the guys afterward to take their time snowmobiling back to the top of the Tram, and next thing you know, we would be flying down the mountain on the snowmobiles going 80 mph. We never crashed a "sled" doing that, but we did crash a few during the season. It got to the point that we, as a crew, were put on probation and told the next person to wreck a sled would be terminated. Funny thing was that I was the next one who would wreck a sled, but it just so happened, I wasn't on duty.

On a warm day when we were not going to work, I took Schmelly up the mountain to go drink some beer and joyride some sleds. We were buzzing along, and the next thing you know, I went over a little hill and one of the skis came off. I left the sled there and went home. The next day, I called from the bar up the mountain to the mechanic, and nobody had anything to say. I went to work that night, and nothing was said. This would be a good time to point out that finding good snowmakers wasn't easy, so I think they just looked the other way.

Probably the highlight of my snowmaking career came one night when it was dumping snow and they had just groomed Gunbarrel, something they did a half dozen times a year. My crew was having fun skiing the barrel while checking guns, so I figured I would settle in for a little nap. I woke up about two hours later and looked out the door of the snowmaking shack. "Holy shit!" It had snowed about three feet. I got dressed and grabbed my skis. The first guy that rode up on a snowmobile, I grabbed by the collar and pulled close, saying as calmly as possible while exploding at the seams, "Take me up there."

I went to the top of Gunbarrel and saw the guys had tracked up the side of the run where the guns were but left the side under the chair untouched. I used my poles to cross to the other side of the run and remember clearly turning my skis downhill and just cutting two deep ski marks in the powder. I pushed off and floated down the slope. If you can imagine the perfect run—slope angle, surface under the powder, consistency of the powder—everything was just right, perfect. After a couple more runs, the Tram operator came in, and I took a couple of my best skiers and headed to the Tram. Since I knew the Tram supervisor, when I asked him to shuttle us up, he asked, "You got guns going up there?" To which I replied yes; next thing you know, we were on our way to the top of the face.

We were on our way down. It was *heavenly*, pun intended. I noticed the Tram was moving, and as it was passing over, I looked up and was greeted by a Tram lined with ski patrol members glaring down at me. It was customary for ski patrol to "cut" the mountain to make sure it was stable to avoid avalanches. We had taken care of that. A little farther down, I could see my boss's truck pull up. Then his boss pulled up, and about a minute later, pulled away. When I got to the bottom, my boss put his arm around me, looked up the mountain, and said, "What do you think I just got yelled at for?"

I couldn't help but smile. I replied, "Well, if I'm going to get fired, do it now, because that is what it is all about."

Without a word, I walked to the shed, changed clothes, and went home. Before I left, I looked up the mountain and was treated to the sight of perfect s-tracks in the snow.

I went to work that night, and Jake (who happened to have been off and missed it) told me that later in the morning, the trail manager, Martin, commented to my boss in his Swiss accent, "You got some good skiers, YA." Not another word was said.

Another perfect winter was soon to close. I was invited on the Management Party Cruise on the Tahoe Queen. It wasn't my finest hour. I got so drunk, and I think it was at that point that the welcome mat, placed before me in previous years, was rolled up and removed.

I ended up going back to San Jose at the end of summer, so I'll never really know.

My final summer at the marina was spent giving parasailing rides. I called it "human fly fishing." We were using a prototype pontoon boat with a stage built onto the back end and a winch to reel people in and out. My job was to put the harness on people and fly the parachute, then have people step up to the stage, where I would buckle them in. While the boat was going forward into the wind, keeping the chute aloft, I would jump down to the front of the stage and use a lever to let the rope out and fly the customer.

There was a three-foot-long red mark on the rope indicating the end of the line. One day, I had gone to work baked after a couple of days off, and suddenly, the rope was pink. I was confused by this new color, and by the time I figured out pink meant red, I had reeled out all the line. The chute and the customer dropped like a rock straight into the lake.

That scared the shit out of me. That was an eye-opener. This job and its inherent risks may have been beyond my desired liability. I think that was a turning point and a watershed moment in my life. Suddenly, my risky behaviors started taking up space in my mind.

I left out a story from the earlier winter season, when Jake and I were caught in an avalanche. The snow was only knee-deep, and when the cloud engulfed me, I just ran out the side. When I looked back to the middle of the slope, I saw the whole slope was moving, so no harm no foul. But had I fallen and been buried, it could have been deadly.

This sudden awareness of my mortality didn't prevent me from another one of the most awesome things I experienced during my time in Tahoe. One night after a BBQ at the marina, there was a full moon. We decided to take out the parasail boat and take some flights. We went far offshore, and as we came back toward South Shore, the moon was bright and full over Heavenly, and the reflection of the Casino's lights in the foreground was mirrored on the lake. The only thing I could hear was the sound of the breeze passing by my ears. Just like my ultimate powder run earlier in the winter, that moment was the apex of my summers in Tahoe.

I was living with Don's son across the driveway from Don, the one-eyed mechanic I had worked with. My risky behavior with random women was an ongoing concern for Don, and my partying was well out of control. Don was like a dad to me, but the bottom line was, he had a son and I wasn't it. As the summer came to an end, I took everything into consideration and decided that I was no longer willing to take the risks involved with living on the mountain, and it was time to grow up. I earned my real estate license the first year I moved to Tahoe. It had taken three tries to pass the State exam as, at the time, my idea of studying was sitting on the deck stoned, drinking a beer while studying.

My mom was in real estate, and that's where I got the idea that that's how I would make my fortune. I moved back to San Jose, and back with Mom. I went to work at Gibson Properties Better Homes and Gardens. After that didn't pan out as easily as I thought it would, I ended up going to work for friends of my mom who owned Property Pages Magazine. I sold advertising to other Realtors. Since this was a sales job and customer relations, I attended plenty of open-bar luncheons and golf tournaments where alcohol was served (it seemed at every other hole). I was right in my element, being paid to party.

I was still living with Mom when Jim, her most recent boyfriend (from LA), sat down with me one night and questioned whether I should be living with Mom at that point in my life. In his opinion, I should not. Jim is the only "Papa" on my side of the family my kids would ever know. I was too old at this point to consider him a "father figure," but he has always been a role model and mentor.

I ended up moving into a house over by San Jose City College that was being managed by one of my co-workers at the real estate office. At that point, I was still trying to do real estate, but I was making good money at Property Pages, so I was not very motivated. Did I mention being paid to party? That living and work arrangement would take me through my first winter and summer back in San Jose.

Around then, I had purchased an old Schwinn road bike off my buddy Darren. Darren would eventually marry my aunt, and therefore, become Uncle Darren. He was also the person who eventually took me to my first 12-step meeting. Not so fast though. First, I stripped the bike down, then painted and rebuilt it. I started riding the bike around town, and again, got the idea that, somehow, I was and had always been an athlete. Just because I was still partying; lots of athletes partied, right? I came across a charity ride in Monterey called the Waves to Wine for the Multiple Sclerosis Society. I would sign up for the two-day, 150-mile ride, and other than running with the cross-country team in school, it would be my first foray into endurance sports.

This would be a good point to remind you that my goal at that time was to prove to people I could party and still compete. My idea of training was riding around town from one friend to another's, getting baked and drinking beer. I had no idea about biking etiquette and protocols. I didn't own a stitch of spandex. I didn't have cleat pedals or bike shoes.

I showed up in Monterey with my trusty bike, cotton sweatpants, cotton sweatshirt, and tennis shoes. I spent the night on the football field at Monterey Junior College in a pop-up tent surrounded by other participants. I made it the first day 80 miles. That night, there was a pasta feed at the school, and of course, my eye was wandering looking for any available ladies; there were none.

The second day was only 70 miles. My lack of experience was starting to show. At the lunch break at Pinnacles National Park on top of the mountain, I left my bike in the sun. During lunch, there was a loud bang that echoed across the plateau. As the rest of the group looked around in disdain, I soon realized it was my tire that blew out. I was embarrassed, but calmed myself with the thought that I didn't know any of these people, especially the ladies.

Luckily, there was a mechanic with a tube there, and my tire was soon repaired. Did I mention bike protocol? Who knew I was supposed to carry an extra tube and pump and tire-change kit? I was able to finish the ride with the help of a couple of old guys, who were properly attired and kindly let me draft my way 20 miles down the coast in a 20 mph sidewind. Again protocol, who knew I was supposed to take my turns at the front pulling?

When we got to about three miles out, I was made aware of that fact by a nice, young volunteer kid who was pointing us in the right direction. As I rode by, he said to me, "Just three miles." I was so spent that I wanted to get off the bike and punch him, but I knew that would be the end of my ride so I smiled in appreciation and rode on. Upon finishing the race, I felt an overwhelming sense of accomplishment. "See I could do it!" Live my lifestyle and still achieve greatness. It would be at least another ten years before I did another endurance event.

Back at the house in San Jose, the ex-girlfriend of the guy who I lived with in Long Beach had moved in. Strictly platonic. Partying at that point involved beer, pot, and coke. Her boyfriend was a small-time coke dealer. One night, I went to Tahoe for a night of partying with Shawn #2's brother, just to break in his new car. I ended up running into Veronica at the nightclub at Caesar's, and since I was no longer "local" and had been classified as *Shy Shawn* with friend status, I was given the stalker treatment as I tried to pursue her all night.

By six in the morning, I had lost my ride. I had 20 bucks left in my wallet. A bus ticket home was $30. I decided I had three choices: (1) Go put $20 on one hand of blackjack. (2) Plead with the driver to let me on for 20 bucks (but if I did this and he said no, I wouldn't be able to sneak on). (3) Sneak on. I decided to go with option three. I walked around the back of the outside of the bus, and when the driver went to the front to get a ticket from another passenger, I snuck onto the bus quickly, sat down, and covered my head with a sweater. It worked, before I knew it, we were down the road heading to Stockton. I made it.

Not so fast, we got to Stockton and some people got off and some got on. The driver did a head count and realized he had an extra passenger. For a split second, we made eye contact, and I swear he knew it was me. I detected a microshake of his head, and he went back to his seat. We departed for San Jose.

When we got to San Jose, I still had the $20 in my wallet, so I could afford and got a cab home. Exhausted both mentally and physically, I went straight to my room and slumped into my bed. It was about ten. I let out a big sigh of relief; I'd made it. After about 15 minutes, my roommate came in and invited me to go with her and her boyfriend and a few of his friends to the Bay with his speedboat. I couldn't help but think *it's not how you feel but how you look,* so off I went.

The coke, Jägermeister, and beers were flowing all day. We hit pretty much every Bayside bar with a boat dock. By the end of the day, I was no less exhausted. I did get the bonus of spending the ride home in the back of the truck wrapped up in the boat cover with Andrea, making out. I would see her once or twice after that, but that was it. When we got home, I went again to bed, glad the 30-hour run was over.

My roommate and her boyfriend had gotten into a fight because of her overindulgence, so he left her behind. About 15 minutes later, I heard the door slam. I jumped out of bed to realize that my roommate was planning to walk the ten miles to her boyfriend's house in the middle of a rough part of town at night. I walked alongside her for a mile, pleading with her to come home, that her parents would never forgive me if anything happened to her. She eventually agreed, and we returned home. Finally, back to the sanctuary of my bed.

Ten minutes later, the doorbell rang. I shot up out of bed and got to the door before her. I opened the door and found it was a cabdriver. I wished her, and him, the best and waived as they drove off. This time I was able to go to bed for the night.

CHAPTER 4

Onward and Upward —Go North

After a hard summer of partying, including late night calls to the limo company (better to spend $200 than drive drunk), it was time for my next move. There was also the fact that my roommate and I had not paid a dime in rent. I was still working for Property Pages and doing well enough financially to get my own apartment. It seems ironic, but I moved to an apartment that was next door to a kid, Kris, with whom I had played Little League baseball. I would have made the all-star team that year, but he made it instead, I believe, because his dad was the coach. As you'll find out later in the chapter, I did get the last laugh.

At the time, Kris was dating a girl named Gretchen. I was dating a girl named Tracy, who, I found out later, was not dating me exclusively. On Halloween, Tracy and I had gone out to a Halloween party and ended up at Kris's apartment playing cards with Kris and Gretchen. Gretchen and I had what I would best describe as an antagonistic relationship. Later, when Tracy and I got back to my apartment, she told me she thought that that antagonistic relationship was more one of sexual tension and that we would end up getting married. I laughed my ass off at that thought. Turns out Tracy was right.

Things were stressful at Property Pages, with deadlines and all, so when I was offered a job with a company selling marketing tools to Realtors, I pounced on the opportunity. The theme of open-bar luncheons and golf tournaments with flowing booze continued. At one point, the company I was working for sent me to Gaithersburg, Maryland, to take pictures of houses for a month. Let me get this straight: I drive around a town I've never been to and take pictures of houses? Hell ya, I was in. Of course, I went with the best intentions in mind. Nose to the grindstone, sobriety, you know the routine. Then of course, the short-term apartment I was staying in was right next to a mall that just happened to have a seafood restaurant that had live music four nights a week and an all-you-can-eat, champagne brunch on Sundays.

Now I don't want to toot my own horn (and I have no idea what it was like before I got there), but it seems to me that with the presence of the crazy dude from *Cali* and his insistence that the DJ end every night with Jane's Addiction and Frankie Goes to Hollywood, business seemed pretty healthy when I left.

By the end of my trip, Tracy broke up with me and informed me that she would not be picking me up at the airport. I had developed a friendship with this girl who was sweet and innocent, and she agreed to pick me up at the airport. By the time I had poured myself off the plane and then let loose my drunken ranting on the way home, that was the end of that friendship and any romantic aspirations toward her I'd had.

Upon my return, I found my reputation as a drunk had preceded me—between the stories relayed back from Maryland and the luncheon-and-golf-tournament circuit—so another change of jobs was in order. Being no longer financially independent, I moved from my apartment and into the condo my mom owned (the one where Jim had asked me to grow up and move out of, some time ago). It was now being rented by Charlie, a dude ten years my senior that I had met through my mom years earlier.

At this point, I took a couple of part-time jobs. The first was working at the Shoreline Amphitheater serving beer—a kid in a candy store. The second was teaching one of those comedy traffic schools. I can say that I have taught at both Berkeley and Stanford. Charlie worked for a pharmaceutical company out of Texas as a sales rep. He set me up with the sales manager for an interview that I blew when I was asked the old question "what is your biggest weakness?" to which I replied, "I probably drink too much." That is probably not the best answer to that question, and I did not get the job. In retrospect, with the amount of travel required and all, it would not have worked out. But the realization that I had a problem was starting to set in.

One day after work, I went to visit Kris, and Gretchen's sister was there watching the apartment. I went back a couple of days later, and Kris told me that he had gone away to a cabin in the mountains with another girl. He did not tell Gretchen, although she had her suspicions. They ended up breaking up, and when Kris told me that, I went straight home to track down and call Gretchen's number.

She told me later that she had told her mom she didn't want to talk to anyone, especially "Shawn." We ended up talking, and we went on a date within the week. We were married six months later. When I met Gretchen's parents over dinner, I told them I was an alcoholic. Again, probably not the best lead, but obviously the truth was setting in. Gretchen was not my "typical" type, but I felt more relaxed and able to be myself around her than I ever had before.

Soon after we married, I got a job offer from my friend's dad in Long Beach to go back to work for the property management company, this time selling management services. Gretchen and I ended up moving to 60 Ximeno Ave in Belmont Shores. Although it was staggering distance to the world-famous Yankee Doodles Bar, I was too cheap to pay those prices for drinks and spent most of my time drinking at home or on the beach.

G. and I would go to the beach and play catch with the football or play Roller hockey in one of the parking lots that was blocked to traffic. We used to smoke pot all the time and drink about a twelve-pack most weekends. I would drink during the week, usually six per day. Gretchen's plan to get me sober was to drink beer to beer with me to keep me from drinking too much.

After having some success at the sales job, I decided I just didn't like the pressure of sales. I was offered a job, through my mom's Jim, at a Statewide Pest Control Company, the one with the little man and the hammer logo. I felt that it was honest, blue-collar work, and I knew I would get paid for my work, something that is not always guaranteed with sales. My original route was downtown Long Beach, and from Wilmington down to the Palos Verdes Peninsula. Since the company was statewide, a transfer to Santa Barbara came up, and I pounced.

Once again, it would be a chance for a geographical move and to leave my addictions behind. G. and I moved into an apartment on the mesa overlooking the Pacific Ocean. My sobriety was short-lived, and I soon found a pot dealer and was in business. I was still drinking only six beers most days and a little more on the weekend.

I finally went to a psychologist, assuming if I could just properly treat my (undiagnosed at that point) bipolar disorder, my addiction would disappear. I soon was prescribed Wellbutrin and Depakote, and things got better, but the addiction didn't go away. My drinking started to escalate, and G. was trying to go beer for beer with me, so I just started buying more.

I went back to school at Santa Barbara City College. Even though I was drinking and smoking, I had a dedication to school and did my best to not miss any class time. I was taking a class, "Cinema as English." We got to watch a movie every Monday night, starting with *A Trip to the Moon*, and progressing through time to some modern movies. I would get drunk and stoned, and I got to watch a movie—best class ever. I did my final paper on the '70s version of *Blade Runner*, and I got an A. That paper, like this book, inspired me to some of my best writing.

I had a catamaran sailboat down on Leadbetter Beach and would go sailing some days after work. One day, my brother-in-law was visiting. As usual, the day started out with light winds, so we started throwing back beers. Then in the afternoon, the wind came up, and filled with liquid courage, I took him out sailing. It was blowing about 30 knots by then, and we were in over our heads. We took a tach away from the beach and were starting to fly the hull. On the way back, he was sitting in front of me. We were flying the hull going so fast that he slid forward and ended up on the front of the trampoline platform.

We promptly did a *pitch pull,* which means we cartwheeled the boat. Mid-flip, I was launched back first onto the mast, and all I heard was POP; I thought for sure I broke my back. I thought to myself, *damn, that didn't feel so good.* Just then, I flipped over backwards and landed headfirst on the hull of the boat. *F*^k, that didn't feel so hot either!* I had been flung out of one of my water shoes, and one of my toes was bleeding (here, Sharky Sharky).

I must give credit to the Harbor Patrol; they were right on the scene. Of course, being too drunk and proud, I refused their help, and they went on their way. As we were floating toward the beach, I noticed we were surrounded by hundreds of dolphins; they created a very beautiful, calming effect. I have heard that dolphins will protect you from sharks. I love dolphins.

Once again, my life was spiraling out of control. Eventually, I was able to cross the stage for graduation at City College, although I was supposed to finish one more class, which I never did. I lost my desire to work in the bug business. I had been promoted to supervisor and found that the stress of (once again) not being able to control outcomes based on other knuckleheads' actions was too much for me. So I chose to search out another job.

Aside from my specialized skills in other fields, I had only general experience in sales, so I took a job as a recruiter for a private technical college. My job was to go into high schools, do presentations during the day, and meet with parents and students at night. Because of the hours, the driving, and the escalating partying, I was not doing well at that job. I decided that, after just a couple of years in Santa Barbara, it was time for another geographical move.

This time, G. and I bought a house in Cambria on the Central Coast near the Hearst Castle in San Simeon. Before I moved from Santa Barbara, my head meds were changed to Ritalin and Lexapro. In Cambria, I met with another psychologist, who put me on kalonapin, a barbiturate. I had started crushing and snorting the Ritalin, so between the two, I was basically doing pharmaceutical speedballs.

Since I had moved out of my job territory, I had to change jobs again. I went back in my history and got a job doing ad sales for a Central Coast magazine. That worked well until it didn't. I was working out of San Luis Obispo, so on my drive home, I started stopping at a bar on the coast in Cayucos. I would get home already launched on my way to my daily buzz.

G. was losing patience with me, and we started moving in different directions. Eventually, I quit the magazine and went to work at a gym in Arroyo Grande selling memberships. That didn't last long. I quit. I went home and was drinking beer and sitting in the Jacuzzi I had recently bought, when G. got home. The look in her eyes said it all; it was all but over.

That weekend, she decided that for the first time during our marriage, she would drive to her parents' house in Sonora by herself. I believe that is when she decided it was over. I spent the weekend at home alone getting drunk. I also did some electrical work. There's a winning combo, drunken electrical work. At one point, I was wiring a dishwasher and there was a small puddle and I saw "the blue flame of death." That could have been the end.

That day, during the Daytona 500, Dale Earnhardt hit the wall and died. When G. got home, I was expecting her to console me, *and that was going to happen.* G. was in no mood for me, and I ended up telling her, "F*^k you, I'm leaving in the morning." I think that helped G. get her desired results, and in the morning, I grabbed my portable TV, my afghan blanket, and my Glock 9 handgun, and left.

I decided I would drive home to Mom's in San Jose, and she would help me find a rehab. When I got to San Jose, I picked up a six-pack and headed to her place. I finished the six-pack waiting for her to return home. When she arrived, we headed to a rehab my sister had gone to in the Santa Cruz Mountains. When we stopped at a gas station to get gas, I ran into the store and bought a 32 oz beer. When we got to the rehab, we were told there were no beds. We were directed to a couple of other facilities, and every time we stopped, I grabbed another beer.

Eventually, we ended up at my sister's house, and I was loaded. She got on the phone, and as I stood there, she hung up the phone and told me if I wanted help that day, I would have to threaten to harm myself. I looked at her and said, "What the F*^k? Fine, I'll blow my brains out." (I had no intention of hurting myself.) She looked over my shoulder, and I turned to find a cop and an EMT standing at the door.

I was *5150ed* (the police code for a person potentially harmful to self or others, earning one a 72-hour stay in a rubber room) and taken to the hospital for a 72-hour hold. I was taken from the ER to the psych ward around midnight and taken to a room. This wouldn't be the last time I was drunk, but it was absolutely the beginning of the sobriety process. Since I came in late, I could sleep in that first morning. That was the last luxury exception I would be extended for the next three days.

Once I was awake, I had breakfast and found the phone. Still hung over and deep in a fog, I found a phone and called G. I was greeted with a coldness I didn't understand, and again deep in a delusional state, I asked her when she was going to come visit me. She replied "never." And that was that.

It was during my 72-hour stay that I attended my first 12-step meeting. After being released, I went home to Mom's house, and for the next 30 days, I attended a half-day outpatient program at the hospital, and 12-step meetings most every day. As I said earlier, Daren had taken me to a few meetings and gave me my first Big Book (Alcoholics Anonymous). Gretchen filed for divorce. She moved from our Cambria house to San Luis Obispo, and we listed the Cambria house and the Santa Barbara condo for sale.

After my 30-day program, my mom was going on a cruise, and I had made a call to the pest control company in Santa Barbara. They were willing to take me back. So again, we parted ways, and I headed back to Santa Barbara for what was supposed to be a life of sobriety. Gretchen and I met up in Santa Barbara and went on a couple of dates, and I went to San Luis Obispo to see her. Although we were intimate every time, things were not going to go back the way they were. On my visit to her apartment at the end, I could tell she was conflicted. I was leaving anyway, so on my way out the door, I kissed the cheek when the divorce was final.

I have not heard from nor seen Gretchen since then. She got a lawyer for the divorce, and I didn't. We sold our homes and paid our debts, and we both walked away with about $50K. I don't know where she is now, but from the minimal searching I've done, I think she used the money to get her master's in psychology and get a job she'd always dreamed of. She lives in a town that is the last place I would have guessed. I have no hard feelings toward her and wish her nothing but the best. If I ever see her again, I have no intentions other than to be cordial.

CHAPTER 5

The Beginning of the End

After eight years married to Gretchen, four geographical moves to different cities, six different jobs, 72 hours on a 5150 stay, and 30 days of rehab, I found myself back in Santa Barbara doing pest control. This was probably one of the most difficult times in my life. Having been recently divorced and through rehab, I felt like an outsider, completely alone. I felt like people just knew I was flawed. I didn't have to say a word to anyone. They just knew.

I moved into a 700-square-foot studio apartment. I still had a large sectional couch and my king-sized bed, so the only way to get from the kitchen to the bathroom was to squeeze sideways around the furniture. There were times I was so full of angst that I would feel like beating my head against the wall in the shower just to make the pain stop. It was at that point that I became the most spiritual I had ever been. I would do my daily devotions, and although they would not eliminate the pain, it helped me to better keep things in perspective as to what true pain was.

Santa Barbara is a college town, so there were plenty of students living in my building. I felt like the old-man outcast. I hooked up with my pot connection, who still lived right where I left him years earlier.

Although pot had been my drug of choice for years, I rationalized that alcohol was my problem, not pot.

I was assigned a route in the Santa Ynez Valley. Each morning, I checked in at the office and drove over the mountain highway 146 from Santa Barbara to Santa Ynez for the day of work. In the evening, I attended 12-step meetings. I was desperately trying to connect with anyone, though I still didn't want to be "one of them." Since I was going to the meetings stoned, it was probably my fault I was having a hard time making connections.

Summer passed, and I started to emerge from my fog. As I mentioned earlier, G. and I had a couple of dates, but that ship had sailed. Then it happened. At the time, I was into coffee. Most mornings, I drank coffee in the office and on my trip over the mountain to Santa Ynez. One time, I had to relieve myself, so I went to the only public restroom in Solvang. After I finished my business, I exited the restroom on the side of the building and saw a sign for "Hot Coffee." I thought more coffee was a good idea.

I walked in the front door, and on the opposite side of the room, a girl came through the swinging doors from the kitchen, walking backwards. Her long dark hair and light brown skin riveted my eyes when she swung around to face me, my heart melting at the sight of her smile. For the first time in months, I felt human again. I wasn't feeling very lovable at the time, but right then and there, I thought she was a woman who could love me. I could just tell by the look in her eye and the positive energy flowing from her body.

Adriana and I had nothing in common when we started dating. She spoke very little English and was ultra-shy to boot. I was just at a point in my life that I needed the stability that she represented. Her now-late parents had been married to each other since they were teens, and she was the baby of 14 siblings. We will have been married 18 years in 2020, but it hasn't been easy. I started visiting Adi, as I call her, most every day at the bakery. One day, I gave her my phone number and turned to walk out. As I left, one of her nephews said, "Hey, she's not going to call you."

Disappointed, I turned toward the door. But then he stopped me and asked, "Well do you want her number?"

I nodded and collected her number. Now would be a good time to mention that Adi spoke very little English since moving from Mexico years earlier. She originally came with her parents on a visa but stayed past the expiration; she was undocumented when I met her. This started a difficult courtship process.

Adi still lived in a one-bedroom apartment with her parents and married sisters' families. When we went out, there was usually a nine o'clock curfew. As you can imagine considering my checkered past, this was huge change in standard operating procedures. Couple that with the fact that, aside from a few short-term relationships, Adi had never been "with" a man.

After a few months of dating, I went to give Adi a peck on the lips at the bakery, and she turned and presented me with her cheek. Again, not standard operating procedure for me. The culture clash was the only thing I could come up with, and I wasn't sure if I was ready for that much work. I decided not to call her again. But after a couple of days, my phone rang.

"Why you don't call me?" she asked in her broken English.

I ended up taking her out again. Funny thing is, we had both lied about our age, each subtracting two years. I started to wonder about that one night when we went to her brother's birthday party. Adi is the youngest girl and second youngest of 14 siblings, nine of whom lived in Santa Ynez. People were wishing her brother Martin a happy 28th. That is the age Adi had told me she was. A little quick math in my head, and things weren't adding up. It was soon after that I learned the truth, and I couldn't help but laugh to myself. At no point did I really wonder how old she was, but I thought it was ironic that we both felt the need to fudge the truth by the same number of years.

At this point, I still was not drinking but I was smoking. One night, when Adi stopped by after English class at night school, I was stoned. I was hugging her and holding her close, and she looked into my eyes and asked, "Why you eye so red?"

I knew that I couldn't continue a relationship with her living a lie. Beyond my wildest dreams, when she left that night, I took what remained from my ounce of weed and sent it down the garbage disposal. I did something I thought was impossible. I quit pot cold turkey.

I had told Adi I was sober a year, but I'm not sure how long it had been. I made the classic mistake of thinking I was ready to go back to drinking, this time in a gentlemanly fashion. Adi's brothers were all drinkers, Coors Light. I had been a Bud guy up until that point. That first Coors Light went down smooth. Sobriety over, I was off to the races.

The culture clash with Adi was still present to the point where I had to decide whether to marry her or break up. Adriana still lived with her older (now deceased), very traditional mother, so Adi was not allowed to go out later than nine o'clock. She had nieces younger than her that were living it up way more. So, I concluded that I had to make a big decision. Should I stop dating her or do I marry her? Those were the only two seeming options.

There was such a sweet, innocent charm that Adi had, and I just knew at the time she would make somebody a good wife and be a great mother. I don't think either one of us was ready to get married, but we were both ready to be married. I decided to ask her to marry me. It was one of the rare nights Adi had come to my apartment to watch television. In a moment of pure lunacy, I asked her to marry me in what was probably the least romantic marriage proposal ever.

"Do you want to get married?" I asked from the couch. It was kind of ironic that we were in a place were millions of ladies have been proposed to—at wineries, perhaps at some of the vistas overlooking the valley. But I chose the couch; I'll never get a redo on that one.

For some reason, she said yes. It may have been that she was just as crazy as I was. Or that of all her brothers and sisters, she was the only one not married. The Mexican culture has strong family values, and she wasn't getting any younger. I was realizing that most of the women who had the characteristics I consider to constitute a good woman were already married or had a boyfriend by then. I, too, was not getting any younger. They say that men who were happily married get into relationships sooner after their wives die than those who were not happy. I believe this to be true of divorced men as well. When I was married, I was generally happy, just not happily married to G. So, I had decided that Adi was going to be a good wife and a good mother, and I didn't want to let that opportunity slip away.

We started planning a big wedding to be held at the Mission Santa Ynez. The reception would bring out all the bells and whistles, including an eight-piece mariachi band. The first obstacle we encountered was the Catholic church. We met with the padre, and immediately, there were red flags. First off, there was the case of my first marriage. Besides that, although I grew up Catholic, I had converted to Lutheran since my first father in-law was a Lutheran pastor and I related more to their doctrine. The priest spelled out an extended list of obstacles that we, or I, would have to overcome to be married in the mission.

Couple that with the fact that the "crazy" was starting to come out from my family also—if you invite one person, the other one won't come, etc. Typical intrafamily squabbling. Then the cost of this shindig started going through my mind, and I did the thing I felt was best; I took Adi and we eloped. Where did we do this? Lake Tahoe. Where else? The Love Chapel, Stateline, Nevada, (torn down years ago) to be exact. I convinced Adi it was the best thing. At that point, she just wanted to be married and start her life with me. I asked her not to tell anyone in her family until we were at least halfway into the eight-hour drive. I figured that would give us a head start if her brothers tried to pursue us. They didn't.

When we got to Tahoe, we checked into the Honeymoon suite at the Horizon. My mom, God bless her, had arrived before us, gone into the suite, and switched the complimentary bottle of champagne with a bottle of apple cider. I was pissed. I scolded her like she should have just known that I had gone back to drinking, and she returned the bottle of bubbly, which I proceeded to drink myself, since Adi is not a drinker.

The next day, Adi and I were married at the Love Chapel. After the ceremony, we went back to the casino and did what any self-respecting couple would do. We headed to a slot machine, where Adi gambled for the first time, she still dressed in her white dress and I still clad in my suit. I ordered a free beer (Coors Light) every time the cocktail waitress came by our machine.

By dinner time at the Edgewood Country Club, I was feeling no pain. When it came time to order, I had the elk. Since it had become apparent to me that Adi was a picky eater who mostly enjoyed chicken, I ordered her the duck. I devoured my elk and a few Sierra Nevada beers, but Adi just picked around the duck. I would later find out that, in Mexico, duck was considered yard bird, basically above pigeon but below chicken on the food chain.

The cat was out of the bag about my drinking, and my mom seemed OK with it, or at least that's how I saw it. Adi and I headed back to Santa Ynez, and we were not greeted with enthusiasm and congratulations. I had asked Adi's parents for her hand in marriage, in Spanish mind you, but all that goodwill went out the door, since her parents had been in Mexico when we eloped. I'm not sure if I was high up on their list of favorite in-laws after that, but in my usual delusional state, I was able to avoid thinking too much about that.

Since my return to the pest control business, I had always said that if they opened a Reno branch, I would transfer there. Well, turns out they did. And I did. One of the hardest things was telling my boss, Ray, who had been my boss all the time I was in Santa Barbara that, within about six months of returning, I was transferring to Reno. Protocol dictated that you should be at a branch at least a year before a transfer and you should get the blessing of your manager before you interview. I did neither of those things, and the somewhat volatile Ray was not happy, but he eventually gave me his blessing. The company bigwigs knew my intentions, and I think they were happy to transfer some company-blood into their new acquisition.

The next thing I had to do was convince Adi to move away from her family and the only place she had called home in America. I felt guilty as hell, but my selfish desire to return to the mountains numbed the guilt. This time I was doing a reverse geographical move. Instead of trying to run from my addiction, I was running from the 12-step group and starting fresh without anyone's preconceived notions that I was sober.

When moving day came, I gave Adi the option to stay. I didn't want her to stay but I didn't want to be the one that moved her away. I wanted it to be her decision to come. Everything had happened so fast, and I guess I just knew that I was on the verge of ruining her life. I told her to let me get down the road a way and then tell her brothers that I broke it off, if she wanted. She told me that she was not willing to live with the shame and loss of face this would have caused her and preferred to go with me. The contents of our one-bedroom apartment were loaded onto a moving van and on their way to an apartment in Reno, so we said our teary goodbyes to her family, and off we went to Reno.

Having just gone through what was probably my lowest point, I can only imagine that Adi must have been feeling the same way. Just thinking about it now makes me feel terrible. What if we had just stayed? Sure, thing is, I probably wouldn't be speaking to you through this book if we had stayed.

Reno was a difficult time. I was living in Reno where the office was, but my route was in Tahoe, North and South Shore. I would leave for the office at 6:30 in the morning, head up the mountain, and not get home some days until 7 at night. Then I would spend time on the phone since scheduling was left up to the technicians. Adi had taken a job with a housekeeping company that took advantage of her in every way they could. Making it worse, she was being bullied by her co-workers.

Neither one of us lived our best life or enjoyed our time in Reno. But there were two things that came out of this period. Adi was intelligent enough to learn the business model that would eventually be applied, down the road, as the model we have used for the last 14 years of owning our own cleaning business. This has provided me the opportunity to write this book. The second was that our oldest daughter, Millissia, was conceived in Reno and born in Tahoe.

After just three months, we purchased a condo in South Shore. The first time I took Adi to see it, she came out of the upstairs unit, walked down the stairs, sat down, and started to cry. That's how trashed it was. But that's why I got a good deal. With my real estate background, I was able to negotiate a complete rehab into the deal, which was to be completed before the close of escrow. I was proud of myself.

We moved in toward the end of summer. Finally, I was back in Tahoe. But the pest control company started to work on my nerves. Knowing that I had moved to Tahoe, the supervisor started insisting that I come into the office in the morning even though this was not a company policy. Since Adi was pregnant, she didn't go right to work, and I believe she felt as isolated as I had after my divorce upon my return to Santa Barbara. I soon told the supervisor to go stuff it and quit pest control for the last time. I was relieved to be over what I found to be a horrid profession. Still, it had served its purpose and got me through some tough times.

At first, I went to work with Doug, the manager at the marina from years ago. Doug and his wife owned a real estate company in South Shore, and I went back to "trying" to sell real estate. If I wasn't out showing property, I was expected to be in the office answering the phones. There was no pay unless I sold something. Again, I found myself engulfed by the stress of a sales job. One day, I went to Horizon, the casino where Adi and I had spent our honeymoon, and applied for a job. I ended up getting a job in VIP Services and soon left the real estate business, again, not for the last time.

Soon after I started in VIP Services, I was able to get Adi a job in the housekeeping department at the Horizon. Where I was treated as royalty, Adi once again found herself being bullied by her co-workers. At one point, she went into the cafeteria, where food was provided for workers. Being pregnant, she went to grab a snack and was told by the cafeteria worker she could eat only once a day. Now that may or may not have been a policy, but I know I used to eat multiple meals, frequently. I went straight to the executive chef, who then informed the worker that, since Adi was pregnant, she could eat as often as she liked.

Believe it or not, I once even earned Employee of the Month. My name was etched on a plaque that adorned the wall of the underground employee area of what was once the great Sahara Tahoe, often frequented by the likes of Elvis Presley. The VIP room had a refrigerator stocked with beer. Nights when I closed, I would help myself to a beer or two while counting out my till. Since my mom and Jim were high rollers, they were invited to parties and comped rooms. As the family member who brought them in, many other workers looked the other way as I attended parties with them, most of the time, getting pretty liquored up. Just like at Heavenly earlier in my life, I believe there were other employees who resented the fact that I got away with thumbing my nose at company policy.

Lord knows, I thought I was having fun. In all actuality, it was just more of the same. I think it was around this time that Adi began to realize that I had a drinking problem. Her brothers were all problem drinkers, but nothing like me. For the first time, she started asking me to control my drinking and began getting embarrassed by me in certain situations.

When my friend told me about a job opening that was going to become available in the group sales department, I thought it would be my dream job. With an executive job in Tahoe, I would be able to buy a bigger house for my growing family. However, things went sideways, and somehow, I was talked into taking a job at the front desk as a supervisor.

It was probably my ego that got the best of me. I was provided a mobster-style, pin-striped suit and I strutted through the hotel like a madman. Problem was, I was freaking miserable. By the time my dream job in group sales became vacant, I had hardly served enough time at the front desk to qualify for another transfer. Besides that, my reputation as a heavy drinker put the kibosh on that opportunity.

I had a little business to take care of. I was scheduled off on Tuesday and Wednesday. That previous Friday, the doctor had informed us that the baby was due, and we could induce any time. Since I was working a day shift Monday, I asked him if we could induce Monday night and leave the hospital by Thursday. The answer was yes, and all systems were going. Millissia was born at 10:00 a.m., February 25, 2003.

This was probably the only instant, other than the moment I met Adi, that I felt my life was normal. A calm came over me, like I was anchored at last. I had a clean slate starting out as a dad. At that point, I knew it was time to quit drinking, that my whole life had just taken a positive turn, and that was my goal. Still, the fact that she was just an infant and (as far as I knew) couldn't tell I was drunk, delayed my attempt to quit.

I was able to grin and bear it through the summer, making it through at the front desk. The highlight came on July 4th, when I was able to get my mom and Jim a ninth-floor balcony room overlooking the lake for the fireworks. I was also given the day off and allowed to attend the 4th of July, VIP pool party. I can remember the look of disgust and concern of some of the bigwigs while I was getting my booze on. The highlight of the day was the fireworks, which was off the hook. Adi, who had to work, showed up at the end of the fireworks just in time to drive me home in the crazy holiday traffic on Tahoe Blvd (Highway 50).

After serving my time at the front desk, my next opportunity presented itself. The part-time host worked at a local radio station and informed me they were looking for a sales rep. I had had my fill of long, irregular hours and was ready to move on. Adi had moved on to housekeeping supervisor at another hotel, so my time at the casino ended. I was probably more of a drunk than when I started.

I went to work selling advertising for the radio station, and it didn't take long for me to remember that I hated sales. Couple that with the restaurant next door, where I would pop in for the occasional cocktail during business hours, and the increasing number of days it was getting harder to get out of bed do to *hangover*, and I wasn't long for that job.

In the interim, I had written and voiced a few of the commercials I had sold, and I enjoyed that.

Adi and I had sold our condo in less than a year in a very hot market and made $80K. We moved to a two-bedroom apartment near the lake, just down the street from where Katie and I used to live. One day, while Adi was at work, I was drunk and out of beer, so I left Millissia in her crib sleeping, with a fire burning in the potbelly stove, and rode my bike to the liquor store. The roads were icy with a recent snow. Between that and my drunken condition, I'm lucky to have made it back. I have done plenty of stupid things, but that was right at the top. I concluded that I was not living the Tahoe life I remembered from when I was younger. Who could? Right.

That Thanksgiving, we took our daughter to see Mom. Upon seeing her, Millissia spun and grabbed me around the neck and did not want anything to do with my mom. I knew, right then and there, what had to be done. I had to make a decision that took into consideration the feelings and desires of someone other than myself.

It all changed one day with a visit to my mom. Adi and I had to have a babysitter for Millissia three days a week. After the four days off, Millissia was so excited to see the babysitter. That day when we went to visit mom and Millissia spun around and grabbed my neck when I went to hand her to Grandma didn't sit well with me. Thinking more about my mom and my child, I decided to give up on my desire to live in Tahoe and do the most mature thing I would ever do, and we moved to Brentwood. At this point, the real estate market was good in the East Bay community of Brentwood where Mom had moved to. The town was growing like a weed, and Mom felt a housekeeping business would do well. So, I loaded up the truck and we moved to Beverly, wait, I mean Brentwood.

CHAPTER 6
Mid-Life Crisis

Once again, I found myself living with my mom, but this time, I was with my wife and child. I went to work at the local Coldwell Banker Real Estate office, where my mom was working as an assistant for an agent named Bryce, as his buyer's agent. In the real estate business, leads are classified as A-leads (the best) to D-leads (the worst). Bryce started by giving me his C- and D-leads to follow up and pursue.

I found myself calling a lot of people who really didn't want to hear from me. This was very discouraging and tedious work. I once asked Bryce why he couldn't at least kick me one or two A- or B-leads a month, just so I could feed my family. His response was, "Why would I do that?" Bryce always fancied himself a strong Christian man, and I found his answer to be somewhat in conflict with those beliefs.

One day, when I was working the floor, which is what we called answering the phone and helping walk-ins, we had some clients walk in. I took them out to show them property. The next day, Bryce had me working with some buyers on a property he was selling. For legal reasons, he didn't want to represent both sides, so he assigned the buyers to me and sent me to get a contract signed. When I returned, Bryce was in the inner office with my walk-ins from the previous day. I thanked him for his help and took over. When I stepped out of the office for a moment and thanked Bryce again, he told me that since I was his buyer's agent, he would be getting half my commission for that deal anyway, so he was glad to help. I was livid. That ended my time as a buyer's agent for Bryce.

While I was settling into the Brentwood real estate market, Adi had started cleaning house for a couple of the agents in my office. Sarah, Joan, and Lynn were the start of the business that would lead to where we are today. I recently learned that it takes a good team of three to start a business—the entrepreneur, the manager, and the artist. I was the entrepreneur with the vision and drive to start the business. I was also the manager, charged with properly completing the paperwork and getting proper permissions. But the most important is the artist, the one who puts her heart and soul into the outcome and is judged a success by results based on customer satisfaction. This was Adriana's role, and still is to this day.

After we started the cleaning company, the business grew from one customer to the business it is today. Having grown up poor, Adi puts her heart into every job like her life depends on it. Her personality is one that people gravitate toward when she does an estimate. Most importantly, people trust her. This is where I am going to inject that when I think of the American Dream, I think of my wife, Adriana. This is also where I must admit that this entitled American has been given my American dream by an immigrant.

Things were okay at Mom's, but they started getting tense early. I was drinking heavily most days, and after finishing my beer, I would get into their wine. This didn't go over well with her and Jim. One night, I was so drunk that I threw up along the side the bed where I was lying. I had to get out of there sooner rather than later. I started looking for a house for my family. With the money left over from the sale of the condo in Tahoe, I had cash for a down payment. Bryce had a condo in a shabby part of Brentwood he was selling, and I went in contract on it. During the home inspection, the inspector crawled from under the house and produced a small piece of PVC pipe.

"This is what the house is plumbed with," he explained. "This piping has been recalled."

When I asked if he thought I should cancel the deal, he said, "If it was one of my kids, I would tell them to cancel."

So, I did. Bryce was not too happy about it, but at that point, I was able to find the courage to stand up for what I thought was best for my family. In retrospect, I am very glad I made that decision and followed through with it. I went on to find a nice, affordable, little three-bedroom, two-bathroom in a good area, and that was my first house in Brentwood. It was all fine and dandy, except the house backed up to a street that was one lane when we moved in but, because of the town growing, became two. I soon found myself squirming through the night as loud trucks and motorcycles raced by.

In order to convince Adi I was doing something to curb my drinking, I started attending a few 12-step meetings. But I still wasn't totally convinced I had a problem. After meetings, I would stop off to pick up beer on my way home. I had settled back into the real estate scene of golf tournaments flowing with alcohol, and martini luncheons, and trips to the horse track. In all actuality, it was the only part of the real estate business I liked.

I can't really tell if I sucked at real estate because I hated it or hated it because I sucked. All I know is that then, as always, I was miserable when I was in real estate. That also led to the question of whether I drank because I was miserable or was miserable because I drank. All I knew was that drinking had morphed from something I used to enjoy (I thought) to a necessity to help change the way I perceived reality. I was going through life doing what I thought I was supposed to be doing, but the inner struggle between the grown up and the child within was destructive. I went on appointments with clients, and all I could think about was that, at the conclusion of the appointment, I would drink to celebrate or commiserate. Either way, I was going to drink.

The cleaning business was growing, and I was seeking just enough real estate work to pay the bills. Then, I was offered a position with another local company as an agent recruiter. This came with a base pay of $1K a month and an expense account. I found myself taking other agents out for two-martini lunches. I was getting paid to participate in the social aspects of the real estate game. The stress of the job soon got to me, though. I found myself great at socializing, but terrible at convincing people to switch companies. Soon I was no longer doing recruiting and was just selling real estate again.

To blow off steam, I started riding bikes on the weekend with a couple of friends and rode by myself during the week. That's when I convinced my friend Gary to join me in entering that year's Bethel Island Triathlon. As I have mentioned, I had always wanted to do a triathlon, and the opportunity finally rose before me. I was training more on the bike than anything. I was counting on my past as a swimmer to get me through the swim and my conditioning on the bike to get me through the run.

On the morning of the event, I suited up in a wet suit left over from my days in Tahoe. All the training I had done up to that point still didn't make that suit any less tight. I had put on around 20 pounds since it last fit. At the start, I went out too fast and lost my breath. Combine that with the fact that I was surrounded by a couple hundred human beings who were kicking and flailing. It launched me into panic.

Eventually, I was able to settle into the breaststroke and to establish a level of calm through some focused breathing. I got through the race, finishing last, and was put to shame by Julie, who I knew from the real estate business. That week, in the local paper, there was a comic illustrating a couple of beer-belly, t-shirt-and-shorts-wearing yokels with Adonis-like men running in the background, captioned "Weekend Warriors." I'm pretty sure they were talking about me and Gary.

I heard about an organization called Team in Training, which helped you train for an endurance event and gave you a paid weekend vacation if you raised money for the Leukemia & Lymphoma Society. Years earlier, my mom had been diagnosed with leukemia, and I decided this would be a great opportunity to raise money for a good cause and do a triathlon. It would also give me a reason to slow down my drinking.

I started training by following a schedule provided by the coach assigned to our Bay area team. Training consisted of biking three days a week, running three days a week, and swimming three days a week. That did mean days with multiple workouts. With my schedule, I was able to do most of my training during the days and drink beer at night. My adage, "Train hard, party hard," was in full bloom.

I got together with the team a couple of times to train at Heather Farms and Aquatic Park in San Francisco. The triathlon I was going to do was the Big Kahuna Half Ironman in Santa Cruz. At the time, my combination of ignorance and belligerence didn't prompt me to question whether a half Ironman was the only, or the appropriate, distance. I was familiar with an Ironman, having grown up with the Wide World of Sports coverage of Julie Moss's iconic finish, and later, from following the Iron War between Dave Scott and Mark Allen, and I could not forget to mention Team Hoyt. During that summer of training, I did do an Olympic distance triathlon at Shadow Cliffs Park, but the accomplishment was lost on me since it was just a training run for the half Ironman. Since then, Olympic distance has become my usual distance.

After training all summer, the weekend of the event arrived. It was the weekend after Labor Day in September. Accommodations were provided at the Dream Inn, an iconic hotel on the beach in Santa Cruz. As a kid, I had dreamed of staying there someday. The Dream Inn was right next to the beach boardwalk and all its rides. Adi and I took our daughter, Millissia, over to the boardwalk to go on all the rides. After that, we went to the pool overlooking the beach and Millissia made a little friend, a child of another participant. They had a great time flopping away in the pool.

We went to the team inspirational dinner and pasta feed and heard from some of the survivors of leukemia. It was very inspiring, and I was able to drink only two beers. About four in the morning, Adi woke up and discovered Millissia was running a fever. We gave her medicine and a cool shower but couldn't get her temperature under 103. I was struggling with the decision to scratch from the event and take Adi and Millissia to the hospital or stay and let my mom, who had come on the trip, go with Adi and Millissia. I didn't believe that my being at the hospital would change the outcome, so I decided to go on with the event.

I was feeling strong as I started on the swim out around the Santa Cruz Pier. I was ahead of a lot of people and felt good as I entered the bike portion. But I couldn't help thinking about Millissia while I was on the bike, which made me pedal even harder. On the turnaround of the bike leg, I realized that Julie, from the Bethel Island Tri, was behind me. That and having Millissia on my mind motivated me to push even harder.

Like the bike, the run was also an out and back, with the turnaround by a totem pole at a park in Santa Cruz. I saw Julie behind me again, which gave me another boost of energy. After a few more miles, I had the finish line in sight. I crossed by the side of the Dream Inn onto the beach. Jim was standing at the transition to the sand and told me that Millissia was fine. Relief rushed through my body, and I was finally able to exhale and enjoy the last mile run on the beach. Crossing the finish line was satisfying beyond belief. Tears streamed down my cheeks, and the feeling of accomplishment overwhelmed me. I had finally achieved a goal that I'd had for most of my adult life.

It didn't take long for that feeling to slip back into the fog. As I walked back to the room after having my metal draped around my neck, I came upon a stand on the boardwalk selling what I affectionately came to know as *Big Beers*, 32 oz cans of beer. Coors Light was my flavor of choice. I went back to the room and found Millissia and Adi sleeping in the bed. I sat back and engulfed my first beer. Aaahhh, it was just like the first time. I jumped in the shower, and my whole body stung in pain as the lukewarm water rinsed over my body.

After my shower, I finished my second beer and headed down to the post-event dinner. I was greeted with even more beer. The coach approached me and congratulated me, confessing that he hadn't been sure I was going to be able to make it. Since I had been absent from most of the practices, he couldn't assess my fitness levels. I don't believe it was the level of my fitness, but the level of my desire that got me through that triathlon. A two-mile swim, 56-mile bike ride, and 13-mile run was spurred by my desire to beat Julie and see Millissia. That evening, when I went back to the room, I slept like a baby. After being up the night before with a sick child and getting up at five, and the physical challenge of the half Ironman, I was pooped. I was out when my head hit the pillow.

In the morning, I woke to Millissia watching the end of a movie. The words from the song struck a chord with me: "Everything has a time for changing; even seasons have a time for changing." And with that, the summer was officially over for me. The fog hung low in the sky. The boardwalk in the distance lay silent after closure for the season. I could only hope this meant better things were on the horizon, or at least sobriety.

But things didn't change when I went home. My drinking didn't slow down, and I knew I needed another challenge. Someone mentioned a bike ride in Solvang called the Solvang Century, which would be held in the upcoming March. I made that my next goal. I had done the Waves to Wine 150, over two days in Monterey. Besides that, I had never done more than 30 miles on a Sunday-morning ride with Rod and Gary. I would soon. I started back on my routine of Sunday-morning rides and 14-mile rides three times during the week.

CHAPTER 7

Normalcy at Last

Adi was pregnant with twins, and I decided this time, I was going to do it. I was going to get sober. I started attending 12-step meetings. I also started riding my bike most days for at least 45 minutes. I was preparing for the Solvang Century ride in March. I was struggling with staying sober. Well, I was not staying sober. But I was still training, and the twins were still on the way.

March arrived, and we drove down to Solvang and stayed with some of Adriana's family. The night before the ride, I started drinking with Adi's family, with the intentions of limiting my consumption and going to bed early. I didn't achieve either one of those things. I finally got to bed around midnight, and the six o'clock wake-up time came way too soon. I was probably still drunk.

It had started raining late the night before, and was raining off and on during the morning of the ride. I decided to pull out because of the lousy weather, not because of my hungover condition. The rest of the morning, I tossed and turned in bed, struggling with disappointment with myself for yet another failure. The house we were staying in had a large sunroof. About nine in the morning, I started to hear large hailstones bouncing off the sunroof, alas. Vindication, I had made the right decision to pull out.

Later that year, in September, the twins, Hannah and Heather, were born. This was it—time to get sober. I had continued to train on the bike and signed up for the Solvang Metric Century that fall. Once again, I loaded up the family and headed to Solvang with a goal in mind. I drank a little less and got to bed a little earlier, and this time, I was able to achieve the goal of crossing the finish line.

The following spring, I attempted the Solvang Century again, and again, I was able to finish. Crossing the finish line, I had tears of joy and accomplishment rolling down my cheeks. A hundred miles was a test of every fiber in my body. My neck muscles were terribly strained. My IT bands (iliotibial bands) felt like I was being continuously stabbed by a knife. Mentally, I was drained, and I couldn't help but question, why? All that slipped away and was replaced by the sense of accomplishment when I crossed the finish line.

That would be the peak of my physical accomplishment for some time. I soon slipped back deep into the fog of my alcoholism. My real estate career was wallowing along. I sold a house every now and then, just enough to pay the bills involved with the business. The housekeeping business was growing at a healthy pace, and we were making enough money to pay the bills and live a healthy, middle-class lifestyle. Most importantly, I was able to spend my 20 dollars a day on an 18-pack and two big beers of Coors Light.

This pattern continued for many years. I was starting to show the outward signs of the heavy drinking. My hands started to shake, and I would sweat a lot. I sank into the worst condition of my life, and the health problems would soon follow. The mental obsession of the alcoholism became all-consuming. I would start thinking of drinking as soon as I woke up. Most days, I was unable to get out of bed until ten or eleven o'clock. I wasn't sleeping that long; I would awake at eight or nine but could only lie in bed immobilized for the first couple of hours of the morning.

On most weekends, I would start drinking around eleven. I would often be passed out by six. During the week, I would start drinking around two, and would be out cold by nine. The other aspect of alcoholism is the compulsion that *drunk is never drunk enough.* I would be very drunk and still chug full beers with the belief that that would get me even drunker. At this point, I was just going through the process of working. My lack of ability to concentrate and focus on real estate rendered me incapable of doing the business.

My first medical malady manifested in the form of heart palpitations. It was a Tuesday night. I had drunk a couple of beers and decided to go to a meeting. When I got home from the meeting, I asked my wife to feel my chest as it felt as though my heart was trying to leap out of my skin. We ended up going to the emergency room, and an EKG confirmed that I was in atrial fibrillation. I spent most of the night trying to get back into what is called *sinus rhythm.*

At about four in the morning, the doctors decided they would sedate (put to sleep) me and shock my heart with the paddles to restore sinus rhythm. The thought of this procedure scared the hell out of me, and I started an ongoing negotiation with God. I made the promise to God that, if I could just get through this, I would do my part and quit drinking. The miracle happened around five, and my heart calmed down. Soon after, I was released from the ER, and on the way home, in a cloudless sky, Adi and I observed a single cloud that resembled a man with bushy hair clothed in a full-length robe.

As majestic as that moment was, it was still not enough for me to quit drinking. The next medical malady was anemia. I found myself running very low on energy and getting dizzy upon standing. It all culminated one night, when I got up out of bed to go to the bathroom. I had to prop my arm against the wall just to hold myself upright. Then, I had to spin off the wall and fall forward to return to bed. I finally concluded that wasn't normal and went to the doctor the next day for blood tests.

Later that day, I received a call from the doctor telling me to go straight to the hospital emergency room and get admitted. My blood hemoglobin that was supposed to be between 11 to 13 something was down to 5. I spent the rest of the night receiving five units of blood transfused into my limp body. I spent the next three days in the heart ward under observation, with fears of imminent stroke or heart attack.

Feeling much better upon release, I went straight back to drinking. After a while though, I decided I would again try to quit on my own. At this point, I was taking medication for the irregular heartbeat, and that seemed to be under control. After about six days without a drink, I went to the gym to go for a swim. About 20 minutes into my swim, I went into the wall for a flip turn. Something was off. During the turn, I felt a dizzy sensation, then a nauseous feeling. As I straightened out, I felt a tingling sensation in my left pinky. I got to the end of the lap, and there was a big, dark spot in the middle of my field of vision. I thought to myself: *Did I just have a stroke? Naah.* I did what any good athlete would do, and I finished my workout.

I went to the locker room and could still not see the center of my field of vision. I was able to drive home, and then later, to a prescheduled check-up as my birthday was the next day. The doctor told me he thought it was just an ocular migraine and sent me home with a scheduled appointment to be seen by the eye doctor the next day.

I went to the eye doctor, and they did what is called a *field test*. The test disclosed that I indeed had some vision issues. The eye doctor sent me next door to the optometrist, who also did a field vision test, and immediately checked me into the hospital. A CAT scan would later show that I had suffered some trauma in the right-rear area of my head, the vision region. I spent three days in the hospital, again in the heart ward. I left the hospital with a prescription for Warfarin, *rat poison.*

You would think that I would have gotten the message by now: *quit drinking or die, or even worse, become immobilized or come down with wet brain.* I reconciled all these possibilities and was ready to pay for my sins. I got a flyer in the mail inviting me to a free lunch discussing a prepaid cremation plan. I love free lunch, so I attended and purchased a plan on installment. At that point, I figured it was just a matter of time until I needed the service. My biggest concern was how was my wife going to pay off the plan before receiving my life insurance policy.

Family members started to visit me one by one and implore me to quit drinking. I still wasn't convinced. The next trip to the ER was due to an uncontrollable bloody nose. The combination of the blood-thinning Warfarin and the alcohol led to blood pulsing out of my nose with every beat of my heart. I had been drinking all day and went to the ER around four. By ten o'clock, unable to stop the bleeding, the doctors wanted to admit me to the hospital. I refused.

I had four beers in the garage at home I wanted to finish, and Adi and the girls, who had been in Mexico, were due home late that night. The doctors decided to discharge me against doctors' orders. Of course, I went straight home and downed those four beers. I couldn't talk Jim, who had taken me to the hospital, into stopping for more.

Somehow, I had been able to get a home into escrow, a referral from Church, actually. I was set to get paid about $10K, and I was planning on taking the family to Disneyland for the October break. Yet, my drinking had reached what I know now was a peak. I knew I just couldn't live like this anymore.

The original event, way in my past, my baby sister's death, was no longer the excuse. As a matter of fact, it started becoming apparent to me that the life I was living was in no way honoring her. To top things off, my oldest daughter wrote me a letter telling me how embarrassed she was of me and how she hesitated to bring friends home after school in fear of finding me drunk. She also went on to say that if I didn't do something, she would, and I assumed the worst.

It was at that point that I decided to go to rehab at a farm on a mountain close to my home, in the wine country of all places. After a few phone calls, they told me I could come the next day, but I decided to wait three more days. I had been given a chance to go to inpatient rehab years before by my insurance company, but had not been ready to go at the time. So now I would end up paying $13K out of my own money. That was supposed to be Disneyland money, but my kids decided they would rather have their daddy get sober than go to Disneyland.

The night before I checked in, I drank my usual 18-pack and two big beers. When I checked in, they breath-tested me, and I blew .10. Turns out, I had driven there legally drunk and had probably driven many mornings legally drunk. They showed me to the new-client detox room—a small room just off the kitchen reserved for newcomers before being introduced into the main housing.

As the nurse that checked me in turned to exit the room, she asked if I needed anything. I asked for a towel as I was sure I would be crying. Why? I wasn't sure. Was it the life lost to this disease? The time lost with my wife and kids? The potential of what I was sure I could have been, squandered. I settled in, and after a while, headed out to meet the other addicts.

My head was spinning in a fog. How had I gotten here? When did my drinking go from being fun, the life of the party to a problem? Days were spent in rehab waking up around six. Most everyone else woke up around seven, but since there were only three showers for everyone, I would get up early and take a shower. I would head back to my room and do some reading before going to breakfast at seven.

After breakfast, there was time for a phone call and maybe a little news on the TV before the first "group" at 8:30. We were limited to about 30 minutes of news first thing and before lights out, and phone calls were allowed only during breaks. Getting on one of the three pay phones was not always easy. There was a full-time cook on duty. He was between cook and chef, and the food was excellent. Sundays were family day, and the families were able to join us for lunch. The TV was left on during the day, and we would catch a little football. It was always tough around two o'clock when the families had to leave, and we went straight to a 12-step meeting after they left.

After 30 days, I was released with my sobriety chip. I was able to go trick-or-treating with my kids for the first time in years, sober. I was very grateful and humbled. The only problem was, I wasn't done. I drank one big beer one night, and then, two the next. Saturday rolled around, and my kids had softball practice at ten, in the park by the am/pm. I dropped the girls off and had already been planning to go buy beer. I did buy beer and put it in the back of my truck and hoped the girls wouldn't see it.

I got home and hid my beer in the usual places, the freezer in the garage, behind the garbage cans. I proceeded to drink in my covert way. At one point, I determined that my family must know what I was doing, and since they didn't say anything, they must be OK with it. Later in the day, I decided for some reason to sign up for Facebook IM. Next thing I knew, I got an IM "hey stranger." It was Katie.

She had long before blocked me on FB and was the last person I expected to hear from. In my drunken state, the raw emotions came pouring out of me. My desire to go back to the good old days of partying and lack of responsibility overpowered the limited judgment and values I had left. My wife was 15 feet away doing the dishes, and my kids wandered in and out of the room during my 20-minute conversation with Katie. After that, I was so drunk but never drunk enough, so I drove around the corner to the store to get two more big beers. I don't recall much else from that night other than guzzling those beers and passing out.

Those would be the last beers I would drink. Since that night until right now, I have never had another drink. I can't guarantee that by the time you read this I will be able to say the same. God willing, I will.

The next morning, I awoke and found my family lined up on the couch. Thinking the day before that they did not know what was going on could not have been further from the truth. I knew, right then and there, that it was not OK, and it never would be. My drinking would never be OK with my family. I had been attending 12-step meetings and working with a sponsor, but I believe it was more apparent than ever, at that moment, my life had become unmanageable. I am not a normal human being when it comes to drink. I was/am an alcoholic.

I met with my sponsor early Monday morning, and as I poured myself a cup of coffee, he turned to me just in time to witness my hands trembling terribly. "Whoa," he said, "what the hell is that?" I broke down in tears and told him, "This disease is kicking my ass."

Just saying those words seemed to put me back in a place of power. I knew I was losing a battle, but most of all, I knew I was in a battle, and at that instant, I decided I was going to fight. I was no longer going to passively sit by and wait for someone to sprinkle magic pixie dust on me or speak some profound magical words. I had to take the battle to this disease, and I was determined to win.

The first thing I had to do was embrace the program and work the program as taught to me by my sponsor the way it was taught to him. It had worked for him and the person that taught it to him. I had to go to meetings every day, sometimes twice. I had to read every day from the Big Book, and I had to establish relationships with other members of the program—they were my lifeline. I met with my sponsor once a week, and we went through the steps.

The program recommends that you come to rely on a power greater than yourself to help restore you to your sanity. I had always had a God of convenience, and it soon became my God of necessity. Somehow, beyond what I was ever able to imagine happened. I was able to start putting sober days together.

The point of sharing my story is not to point out how "special," "unique," "different," I am. Nor am I going to tell you that I was such a hard case that, if I can do it, you can. I don't know what I don't know—your circumstances. I do know that it can be done because I did it, and many others have as well. I honestly hope you don't see yourself in these stories and you do not have this disease. But if you do, if you see yourself in any of these stories, there is hope. You just need to reach out.

CHAPTER 8

The Finish Line
Is in Sight

My journey has consisted of a run at physical and mental redemption. The beginning of my redemption started after nine months of sobriety. My cousin had been asking me to do the Discovery Bay Triathlon with her, so on New Year's Day, 2018, I decided to take her up on the challenge. She told me at the time that she would prefer to do a marathon. I had never done anything longer than a half-marathon during the Big Kahuna Tri, 11 years prior, so I was intrigued. She had done the San Diego Rock 'n' Roll Marathon with Team in Training some years before, and being a supporter of Team in Training (Leukemia & Lymphoma Society), I jumped on the opportunity. I went home that night and signed up online, and it was on.

The next thing to do was start training. I'll go into training more specifically in my next chapter. Suffice to say, I was doing a lot of running. Earlier in the year, I had also come to the realization that, much like admitting to myself that I was an alcoholic was the first step in recovery, this also held true for my real estate career. I realized and admitted to myself that I sucked at real estate and hated it. So I decided that at the beginning of the year, I was not going to pay the $1000 in Association dues for the Real Estate Board, and I was out.

The relief from the realization I didn't have to do real estate anymore and the acceptance and the joy I felt was abundant. I enjoyed the first month or two and ran most every day. The cleaning business Adriana had built was doing well enough to support the family, and I assumed the role as stay-at-home dad. I did still want to contribute to the family's bottom line, but for the life of me, I couldn't figure out what I wanted to be "when I grow up."

It was out on a training run one day when it came to me: *This is what I love to do. Train, be outdoors, motivate and inspire people.* I decided then, I was going to pursue endurance coaching. When I got home from my run, I went to the USA Triathlon page and investigated their coaching certification process. There was a level-I course coming up toward the end of the year in Phoenix. I signed up. I also discovered that the level-II coaching certificate has two paths, one with experience and one with a degree in health sciences. So, I enrolled in online college, and in the first semester, I finished college math and started biology. I also took an English class. I was able to transfer a lot of my college units from Santa Barbara City College and could get my AA (associate in arts) in health sciences in a couple of years.

From the start, biology was very confusing for me. But by the time we got into macronutrients, and eventually, muscle fibers; ATP (adenosine triphosphate), the body's energy source; heart; lungs; etc.; it all became very interesting to me. It didn't take long until I was bitten by the biology bug. Don't get me wrong, I didn't become an A student by any means. But I was able to pass Biology 1 and 2 and learn a great deal. I still am constantly reading about nutrition and training. I started out the year wanting to be a coach, not sure what that would look like, and by the end of the year, after the USA Triathlon coaches' clinic and the Triathlon Science of Sport convention, I knew what it meant and what it would take to be a coach.

April rolled around, and I had decided since I was training, I would do the Discovery Bay Triathlon. I lined up on the dock at the marina for my first triathlon in 11 years. The gun sounded. Since I was a swimmer, I went off strong as I had years earlier in the Bethel Island Triathlon and soon found myself experiencing the same results. I was out of breath and surrounded by hundreds of other flailing human beings immersed in water. I slowed my roll and settled into a nice pace and made it through the swim.

On the bike, everything was going along fine until my bike tire dropped off the two-inch ledge of a shoulder. When I tried to casually turn back up onto the roadway, I was slammed to the ground sideways. I landed on my shoulder and banged my helmeted head. That didn't feel so great. I jumped up, shook myself off, and looked around, embarrassed and hoping nobody saw. They didn't. I was all alone on a long stretch. Problem was, I soon discovered, the reason no one else was around was that I was near the back of the pack, and most everybody had already passed on the turnaround.

The run wasn't much better as apparently my training was not quite up to my ambition. When I was finished, they were dismantling the expo area and my bike was the last one in the racks. I was last place unless you count the gal that crashed and had to be airlifted out. (UPDATE: She spoke at the start of the following year's race; she was fine.) I finished with a time of 4:15:00. Work needed.

After the abysmal showing, my spirits were bolstered with a sense of achievement. I had just passed the one-year sober mark, a feat that I had recently thought of as impossible; so keeping that in mind, I just stepped up my training for the marathon. I loaded up the family on June 1st and headed for San Diego. We stopped the night in Solvang to visit my wife's family. At the family dinner, most of her brothers sat in disbelief that I had been sober for more than a year and that I was going to run 26 miles. The satisfaction I got from their disbelief was enough to make any cravings for beer disappear.

The next morning, we drove to San Diego. After our arrival, we headed to the beach. It was a beautiful San Diego day, and the girls were enjoying themselves in the surf. We had a great time. In the past, I would have been shaking and in a rush to get back to the room to drink, but not this time; it was great. After trying to go to bed early, four o'clock came around fast. In San Diego, it tends to be foggy in June, but this morning, it was clear. The weather turned out perfect, and it was a great run.

My cousin Jodi, being younger and fitter, and having marathon experience, had no choice but to run on without me. At one point, I was dueling with a man in his '80s. I would run past him and then walk, and he would run past me. This went on for about ten miles, but I must admit that microcompetition drove me through that run. At about mile 21, we ran onto a freeway that was a gradual uphill slope for about three miles. The legs were starting to burn and stiffen. With about two miles to go, I knew I'd had it. I could crawl from there if I had to.

Some marathons have a cutoff time so that, if you fall behind, a truck pulls up and invites you in for the ride back. Toward the end, I was glancing over my shoulder occasionally, looking for that truck. I was able to keep enough people to fill the truck behind me, and ultimately, I never saw it. It was a metaphor for my life at that moment; I was running from my demons and fighting my ass off not to get caught.

I finally reached the finish line; my girls were standing at the edge of the fence leading into the finishing shoot, and since I was alone, I grabbed them, one on each side. I have a finish line picture that I will always have engrained in my mind. One girl on each side, and they are both looking up at me with huge smiles and glowing faces. Worlds away from where I was just a little over a year earlier. I finished in 6:15:00, nothing to brag about and somewhat laughable, but everything considered, it will always be considered an accomplishment in my heart.

During this time frame, I continued to train. I tested for and received my USA Triathlon level-I coaching certification, and at the end of the year, attended a USA Cycling coaching seminar, tested for and received my level-III coaching certificate. How ironic that USAT starts at level I and USAC starts at level III. On top of that, the online website I use for coaching gave me a level-II designation. I know, confusing, right? So now I knew what it means to be a coach, what I was supposed to do, and what it looks like. I also learned from USA Triathlon that it is better to be a coach or an athlete; it's difficult to be good at both. So, I decided to build my coaching business slowly and finish up the events on my schedule for the year, then next year, do three triathlons.

After receiving my coaching credentials, it was time to focus on being an athlete. The first event was the Rock 'n' Roll Half Marathon in San Francisco in early 2019. The family and I drove to the city and checked into our room. We headed down to the event expo at Pier 58, and I checked in and got my stuff. We then went to Pier 39 for dinner, where I carbo-loaded with a sourdough bowl of clam chowder. From there, it was on to Ghirardelli Chocolate for $20 sundaes—on the bucket list but consider it done. I counted that as carbo-loading too, although I don't think highly processed sugar counts.

Once again, four in the morning rolled around way too early. It was foggy first thing in the morning, but it was a good day for a run. I had an athlete that I was training running with me, but he was not at my fitness level, so about halfway, he told me to run on without him. I was feeling strong after more than a year of continuous training, so I ran on. We ran over the Golden Gate Bridge (check that off the bucket list). I finished in 2:40:00. That would put me on pace for a 5:10:00 marathon.

I did the Bay to Breakers, another bucket-list race, with my cousin Jodi and Miss Adrianne from church. This run is well known around the world for everything that is San Francisco. Naked people and open consumption of alcohol are the norm. We counted 26 naked men and 3 naked women. The bottle was being passed at the start line, and I kindly declined. I couldn't even imagine drinking and running combined. We did the bonus mileage, making it a 15K and came in at two hours. That was a good run for our group, and you'll notice Jodi didn't run away from me.

After that, it was this year's Discovery Bay Triathlon. I started off the swim with my newer approach of a measured pace. I used the sleeveless wet suit and I was fine. I didn't win the swim, but it was my best swim to date. I had a strong bike and run. I did not finish last and knocked 30 minutes off my previous time, finishing in 3:45:00.

Next was the Armed Forces run in Walnut Creek that started at and included a run through the (usually off-limits) Concord Naval ammunition storage facility, acres of mounds with doors containing who knows what. It seemed like a natural thing to be doing on Memorial Day weekend, and Miss Adrianne and I came in at two hours for 12K; a little off our Bay to Breakers time but good just the same.

My next event for the summer was the Herbalife24 Los Angeles Triathlon. I would recommend this race because, how often do you get to swim in the ocean off Venice Beach and bike on closed roads all the way to downtown LA? Then once in downtown, you get to run some pretty famous streets that are also closed to traffic. I must give a shout-out to my friend Rick Adams, who picked me up at the airport and taxied my rear end around LA; he is a true friend. The worst part of the trip was in the airport for my return. A sixish-year-old kid sat next to me in the terminal, coughing and sneezing, and I was thinking to myself *I hope I don't get sick.*

The weekend after the LA Triathlon was the classic Escape from Alcatraz Triathlon. Another bucket-list race. Unfortunately, my concerns about getting sick had fulfilled themselves. The family and I headed to the city and went to registration, where I picked up my packet. I had my arm-and-leg number tattoos applied and was ready to go. The family and I went to the Marina Beach, and as the kids were swimming, I met another athlete and promised to pick him up in the morning from his hotel and give him a ride to the venue. The girls and I walked to the Wharf for some fresh crab and calamary and headed back to the room. I had already developed a cough, and during the night, when I would cough and breath in, I would get a serious tickle in my throat, causing me to cough more.

I was starting to get concerned. I was thinking the middle of the Bay was not the place to have a coughing spell, so I regrettably decided to scratch from the race. I did get up and give my fellow competitor a ride. Later, after letting the girls sleep in, we headed down to the venue as we still had VIP finish-line passes. We were able to watch the top athletes cross the finish line, and I think my wife had a better understanding of the challenges I face doing triathlon. The winner interview was done right below where we were standing, and the girls ended up on the evening news, so the weekend was not a complete bust. The important takeaway here is that I was not willing to risk the possible downside for an upside that was strictly personal.

A few weeks after missing out on Escape from Alcatraz was the Folsom Triathlon. Starting with a river swim in water freshly melted from the snowcapped mountains above, I went with the full wet suit. The bike was much like where I train—rolling, rural hills. The run was a nice run through the town but spent a good amount of time on a path along the river. As much as I had wanted to get out of the river in the morning, during the much warmer run, I was contemplating going back in. My time was about the usual, so nothing to brag about.

Later on that month, a couple of weeks after Folsom, was the Long Beach Legacy Triathlon put on by USA Triathlon. This was a warm-up run for the course they are going to use during the 2026 Summer Olympics in LA. I must give a shout-out to my boy Ricky, who again taxied me around LA, this time Orange County and Long Beach. I was excited for this event since I had lived in Long Beach years before. It brought back a lot of good memories of time spent on the beach throwing the football with G. and windsurfing in the Bay.

Saturday morning began at four o'clock, and the race started at seven. The swim was in the Alamitos Bay, and since this was a sprint distance, half my usual Olympic distance, the swim went by fast and smooth. The bike was two laps out and past the iconic Queen Mary ship, which (having stayed the night on it once before) I do believe is haunted. The run was on the beach bike path where G. and I used to duel-to-the-death finish on our impromptu bike races back in the day. I finished with a time that, if doubled, would have been less than my normal Olympic distance time. But that just proves we lose energy over time of performance.

A couple of weeks after Long Beach, I was in Cleveland for the USAT Age Group Nationals. I got to sleep in until five o'clock, an hour later than usual for me, and woke up before the alarm sounded. I did my normal routine and headed to the shuttle for transportation. Rolling through the streets of Cleveland pre-dawn in a bright-yellow school bus cranking rock 'n' roll was surreal.

At the start, the swim was determined to be dangerous because of the waves but they did not cancel; they only shortened the course, to 750M. It was a good thing they shortened the swim as I decided to wear my tri suit, which is a skintight suit used for all phases of the event. Since it was skintight, my breathing was labored, and I struggled through the swim. The bike through downtown Cleveland was interesting, and I do believe they found every hill in Cleveland. The run started on the streets, went through some high-priced, lakefront neighborhood, and concluded with a winding run through a park. I finished with my usual time and did not qualify for 2020 Worlds in Edmonton, Canada.

Thus, ends my recounting of my journey of recovery and redemption. It is a never-ending journey and looks different for all people. My redemption is not just about my opportunity to challenge these endurance events. More importantly, it is being at my kids' softball games, doing the dishes for my wife after dinner, and basically being present and accessible when called upon to be a husband or father. As part of my journey, I hope I can model that it doesn't have to take years of sobriety to experience redemption. It can start the first day you are sober, and after that, it never really ends.

CHAPTER 9

Life as a Grown-Up

I mentioned earlier I would cover training. Here we are. I mentioned starting with running, and that is a good place to start. For some people, walking may even be the place to start. Anything to start moving and developing the habit and routine. For myself, I get to the point that my day just doesn't feel complete until I get in some form of a workout. Some days that just means going for a walk after dinner.

Triathlon is known as a multisport endurance event. This means that just running is not enough. I find it is best to do all three disciplines, at least twice a week, so some days you end up doing two workouts. I like to get in a run most days, and at least, one long run once a week. I bike a couple of 10–20-mile rides a week and a 30-miler on the weekend. I have the luxury of swimming 30–50 minutes two or three times a week.

As I mentioned earlier in the book, start with the end in mind. Fitness does not happen overnight, and if it did, it probably wouldn't last because the effort, the journey is a big part of the joy experienced when results start to manifest. We all know that taking care of ourselves is important to living a good life, I think? Having the health to do what you want is vital. But just knowing that is not enough. It's like drinking; I knew it was bad for me, but the short-term reward was stronger than the long-term effects.

So for me, I had to dig deeper into the WHY? I did get to the point where I desired to live longer than the life I was living would probably have afforded me, but again, it's more than just that. When I was drinking, I didn't garner the respect of my family. I felt like crap most of the time and looked like crap as well. When I was younger, I felt attractive and vibrant. Just because I grew older and more mature doesn't mean that I lost my desire to have self-confidence and be attractive. So that is what drives me to find the energy to work out. Results do not happen overnight, but when they start to show up, momentum is gained.

Training involves adaptation to stress. I'm not talking about the stress we feel sitting in traffic or going through the airport, although we do adapt to that kind of stress. The three key stressors involved in conditioning are *duration, frequency,* and *intensity.*

Let me first say that part of the result of our current condition as a society is the constant need for *homeostasis,* the constant desire to be comfortable. There are different types of homeostasis. Inside the body at the cellular level, there is a constant battle to achieve homeostasis. That is good and necessary. But I am talking about the desire to have our environmental conditions achieve a constant. Heat/Cold are environmental stresses that are a necessary form of stress—stressors that cause our body to go through vital biological changes that are part of the constant development of the human organism. Things like cryotherapy or heat therapy or sauna Jacuzzi help the body to regenerate healthy cells, maximizing control of inflammation.

These are all forms of *recovery.* Recovery is a very important part of training. And a very important part of recovery is sleep. Most biological adaptations occur during sleep. I find that a lot of people today wear lack of sleep as a badge of courage. Personally, I don't agree with this sentiment; I think the discipline it takes to properly maintain the body is much more difficult. There are others who simply must make a choice between working out or sleeping. I encourage my athletes not to sacrifice sleep, and instead, to take a long look at where their time is being spent. Do you watch the news for an hour every day? What I don't do is ask athletes to sacrifice time with family. You may have figured by now, after 30 years of drinking, my family is my priority. I don't tell my athletes how to prioritize their lives, but I find it best to work with athletes whose values are congruent with mine.

Training is not a straight line from an axis point of zero, crossing the scale to 100. For training to be effective, one must stress their body physically, then allow adaptation through proper recovery. The line on a chart should be going up and down with the line trending gradually in an upward fashion. As a coach, I know the way to monitor fitness gain or loss or stagnation is using metrics. This is where the online tracking program I use comes in for coaching, scheduling workouts, recording the metrics—duration, frequency, intensity—and quantifying the results in chart form.

Another important factor for training is heart rate. A person can record their perceived exertion and that is important, but the heart rate is not something that an athlete can control. Your heart rate during activity tells the story of the level of stress the body is under. Stress like heavy traffic, when you are trying to get to the airport, raises the heart rate. When we adapt and learn to relax in traffic, our heart rate goes down.

When developing a workout schedule, most follow the typical form called *periodization training*. Workouts are scheduled in a way that maximum fitness is achieved the week of an event. There are four levels of periodization—base, build, peak, and transition—and most training plans occur over periods of anywhere from 16 to 26 weeks; some athletes maintain an annual plan.

As part of training, it is important that athletes properly taper, or slow intensity of training just prior to an event, without giving up fitness gained. A coach must determine the starting point for measure of fitness. This is done with a test of all-out effort over a period of 60 minutes to determine the maximum sustainable heart rate; it can be as short as 20 minutes but may not be as accurate. Once established, this is labeled either *functional threshold power (FTP)* or *functional threshold heart rate (FTHR)*. There are different terms for this level: *anaerobic threshold or lactate threshold.* There is also a simple math formula to determine a figure, but this is based on averages set by others. The important thing to understand is I would not ask a 50-year-old who just came off the couch to try to maintain a 180-beats-per-minute rate for an hour. Heck, ten minutes to begin with.

Establishing FTP or FTHR is very important and should be determined relatively early, but should not be considered a medical stress test. Once a maximum heart rate has been established from the person's training zones based on percentage of max heart rate, this can be established. I use a workout method called a *polarized method.* During any given workout, 80 percent of the workout will be done at a lower heart rate in the established zones and 20 percent in the higher heart rate zones.

Heart rate zones vary from 60 to 70 to 80 to 90 percent of FTHR. Workouts done in the higher heart rate zones are classified as *high intensity interval training (HIIT).* There are plenty of coaches who believe that HIIT is the best way to maximize use of time to gain fitness over shorter time spent on any given workout. For endurance sports, through my research, I have determined polarized to be the most effective method for endurance training, but if only a short amount of time is available for a workout, HIIT is recommended.

Working with a coach involves more than just workouts and metrics analysis. When you are training for an endurance event, the following considerations are critical: nutrition; hydration; what to wear; how to set up a transition area; how to register and check in for an event; what to do the morning of, the weekend of, the week before an event. For the first-time athlete, these are all questions that can be answered by a coach.

Nutrition and hydration are a huge part of endurance sports. Without proper nutrition, you could hit "the wall" and just *DNF.* Did-Not-Finish athletes must manage the consumption of calories during an event *before they are needed*; waiting until you start to feel the effects of lower glucose levels is too late. There are three different fuels in the body that the body uses to move the body, depending on the level of intensity or heart rate zone.

In the case of hydration, an athlete's failure to manage hydration can lead to extreme health issues; even death can occur. Hydration is more than *drink water* or *drink electrolytes*; a combination of the two are necessary. If you drink too much water and sweat out minerals, you can find yourself experiencing *hypernatremia*, swelling of the brain. On the other hand, too much electrolytes and not enough water can lead to dehydration and high blood pressure, increasing the risk of heart attack. Dehydration also leads to the blood getting thicker and more viscous and decreases the volume of blood and diminishes the body's capacity to regenerate red blood cells. This to can lead to a heart attack.

Being an athlete piqued my interest in all this stuff, and I am constantly reading, just learning and absorbing all the information I can. That's where I came up with the name Aging-Athlete Endurance Coaching because that's what I am, an aging athlete. No one can question my qualifications in that regard. I also decided on that name because, aren't we all aging athletes?

The ironies of life always seem to amaze me. The first being that I sit here on the unofficial last day of summer to conclude this book. I also am going to share with you why just when you (I) have things figured out, things change on a dime. Let me start off, though, wrapping up my thoughts on endurance sports, triathlon and marathon to be specific.

I decided to become a coach and immerse myself in endurance sports to achieve the ultimate joy of doing what I believe I was called to do on this planet. I'm talking about a daily activity here. I do believe that there have been specific moments and interactions that were more meaningful at the micro level. Being a son, a husband, a father, and friend has been more impactful at the macro level. But for now, let's focus on coaching.

I decided to take up coaching because I am intoxicated by the joy of seeing someone achieve a goal they had set out before themselves, not knowing in the beginning whether they could achieve that goal.

I believe that, with a little coaching and intentional training, most people can achieve those goals and experience the joy associated with the accomplishment. As a coach, I also garner happiness from seeing people improve their level of fitness. I have read studies that indicate that higher levels of fitness and cardiovascular health can be conducive to living a longer life. Ironically, that is not the number one selling point of coaching or working out; but for me, it's near the top.

The benefits don't affect just the athletes themselves but extend to the people with whom they most come in contact. Their families, I believe, ultimately benefit through this process because a healthier and happier loved one is just a good thing. If I can help spare someone's children and spouse the suffering that my family had to endure when I was deep into my addiction, I consider that a positive. If I can, in any way, help someone live a longer life and be there for their family longer, again gravy. The benefits of coaching are many and the detriments (of any I can think of) few, so most of what I get to do is filled with joy. As an athlete myself, I get to experience all the benefits I have listed for myself and my family.

One of the great things about endurance sports is just being in an environment populated by healthy, good-looking people. Perhaps not so good-looking where I'm involved, but generally. I have found the people of the tribe to be cordial and supportive. When there are rushes of testosterone involved, you are bound to bump up against athletes so focused they can be intimidating, but not standoffish. That's another one of the reasons I chose endurance sport. Though I perceived it to be a little intimidating, with my naïve, make-myself-at-home attitude, I have been able to blend in nicely and enjoy helping others to do the same.

My associations with the USA Triathlon and USA Cycling have been very welcoming and not overbearing. I have had the opportunity to speak freely and openly with the employees, from chief officer to the head of coaching to the people who are involved with day-to-day operations. These people all work at the national level, and some at the international level, but are very approachable.

Overall, I believe that endurance sports are very much participation sports. Don't get me wrong, I do enjoy watching these fine-tuned athletes perform. But trying to watch a couple hundred athletes spread out over a multiple-mile course can be challenging, especially when I am participating and most all the action is well out in front of me. The ITU, or International Triathlon Union, a combination of governing bodies from around the world, is taking steps to make triathlon a more viewer-friendly sport. First, they are designing more courses shorter, with multiple laps that cross in front of viewers more than once. Another innovation is the inclusion of *drafting* in the bicycle discipline. For all events, other than *draft legal,* drafting is not legal, and participants must maintain a three-bike gap either immediately after passing or being passed. This makes for a much more challenging bike portion, and strategy is more prevalent.

There is also a relative newcomer to the world of endurance sports, *obstacle course racing.* Spartan and Tough Mudder are just a couple of organizations in that field. Personally, I am in the process of getting my coaching certification with Spartan and will be attending the world championships in Lake Tahoe at the end of the month, not competing. I will also be attending an "Obstacle Course Specialist" clinic to start the process of learning for Spartan.

Obstacle course racing is growing in popularity and doesn't seem to be going away anytime soon. I am not an expert yet, but from what I have seen, it does seem that because it involves multiple planes of movement, the popularity is growing with a younger demographic. I think you can get hurt running, biking, and swimming. But the odds of injury increase when body movement occurs on multiple planes and axes. As with anything though, I believe good coaching and proper training can help minimize those risks.

My plans are to continue to grow my coaching business and perhaps even create something lasting that contributes to the sport long after my participation ends.

CHAPTER 10

Crossing the Line "Battered and Beaten" but Complete

I started off this final chapter believing that life is full of ironies. Once again, over the last few weeks, I was confronted with the challenges that life can throw at you. It started in Cleveland, when I wrapped up what I believe was a triumphant summer I'd spent overcoming adversities and achieving my goals, and the redemption of completing seven triathlons. First though, I must accept the fact that I was unable to complete my goals as originally scheduled.

I was going to do my second tri of the year at the iconic Wildflower Tri in Central California on my birthday, May 5th. Due to managerial issues with the organization, that event was canceled. I was disappointed, and even a little irked, when I found out that USAT had an event at that venue on that date, but I was not aware of it until well after. Then in June, after the LA Tri, a snivel-nosed tike in the airport exposed me to a bug, and I was sick and had to withdraw from the Escape from Alcatraz Tri. I hope I will get to do it next year; notice I said "get."

Finally, I have decided to withdraw from the Malibu Tri. It boiled down to a money issue, and although I have a very loving, supportive wife, she has grown tired of watching the money flow out, and honestly, flight and room alone was about a thousand dollars. From my perspective though, I am glad to have concluded my triathlon schedule for the year. I do have one marathon in Las Vegas on the strip at night coming up later this year.

That brings me to my next irony, one that is a little more personal. After such a challenging but rewarding season, I was confronted with the joy of completion but also the accompanying letdown of facing where I go from here. The adrenaline rush is over for now. Summer is soon over for now. Every year around this time, I start to have vivid dreams of living in Tahoe and working on the mountain, preparing for ski season. I usually wake up temporarily disappointed and with a heavy heart that it was just a dream.

This year, I didn't help myself. As I shared with you, I have been diagnosed as bipolar and am on medication to control the symptoms. I have been brutally honest with you in this book with the intention of perhaps helping you, whatever your circumstances may be. I will continue to do so. Recently, after returning (what I considered *triumphantly*) from Cleveland at the now end of my season, I decided I was feeling so good I would wean off my meds. I have tried to do this in the past a couple of times, and both times, according to my wife, mother, and children, unsuccessfully.

According to Einstein or Freud or some person smarter than me, the definition of *insanity* is doing the same thing over and over and expecting different results. I am not sure why I am so intent on quitting my meds other than, as an addict, I don't think I should be putting mind-altering chemicals in my body. It's odd, I don't think if I were diabetic, I would try to wean off insulin. Perhaps, too, my desire to stop taking meds is motivated by the diminished but continuing societal stigma associated with mental health issues. The prescribing doctor has even told me that these meds have been around since the '60s, and there are no studies indicating long-term detrimental effects.

As a result of stopping my meds, I was on the verge of filing for divorce from my wife and willing to turn my back on my kids (whose continual bickering didn't help). I even met with my pastor, and upon being given the company line on divorce and parenting and taking care of your parents, I told him I was capable of turning my back on all of that. Did I mention my mom was just recently diagnosed with stage 4 lung cancer? Hence, the "honor thy mother and father" part, as I was finding it difficult to show compassion to a lifelong smoker who apparently didn't read the warning on the pack. Luckily, that's when I concluded, by myself this time, that perhaps weaning off meds was not a good thing.

Although my training partner, Cousin Jodi, figured it out, and my wife, pastor, and mother had their suspicions, I figured this one out on my own. Another glaring red flag was that, for the first time in almost three years, I was considering the desire to chemically alter my perception of reality, and isn't that just another form of medicating? Like I said, life's ironies, am I right? As soon as I figured out things were going haywire, I immediately went back on meds and headed straight to a 12-step meeting. The good news is, damage was kept to a minimum. I have been back on my meds and am back to my normally optimistic self.

More irony. You may have figured out by now that my venture into endurance sports is like a metaphor for my life (Hebrews 12:1 Let us run with perseverance the race marked out for us). I may finish a race, and although not always victorious, I am a survivor. But as soon as one challenge is over, the next one is right around the corner. Maybe a brief time to relax and celebrate, but it's soon time to get back to work. Honestly though, I don't think I would prefer it any other way. Life without achievable goals would be boring. Not ever achieving goals would be disheartening.

For now, I will continue training for a marathon in Las Vegas. Soon after that, the holidays will be upon us, a time to celebrate the triumphs, and then life goes on. If you get this book around the new year, I hope it will help motivate you, perhaps with a resolution either to give up something you have been doing that is harmful to yourself and detrimental to your loved ones or to take up doing something that is the opposite, beneficial to yourself and your loved ones.

Epilogue

This has been the story of my life, condensed. The important thing I wanted you to glean from this is I am not special and hope I have not come off as thinking so. But I am probably more like you than different, so perhaps that makes us both special. It has taken me just a little over a year to write this "addiction memoir" (as one editor put it, and I believe that is a fair assessment).

Who am I to write a memoir? Well, that was just the classification, but what I intended to write was a story. I wanted to be brave enough to shine as much light as I can about mental health and addiction, knowing that it will probably cost me a pound of flesh eventually. I consider myself just another foot soldier in the trenches, and if you feel the same way, just know there is a way out; there is help. Addiction is a disease of isolation, and our enemy wants to get us alone and kill us. If anything I said even provokes a new thought, make sure you get honest with yourself. You are the best friend you have.

About being honest, I have written this based on complete honesty, willing to be vulnerable in hopes it might benefit you. I have been struggling with a dark secret since my trip to Mexico in October. You can probably guess where this is going. I had been missing support group meetings a lot over the summer because of travel doing my event schedule. I started telling myself a month before I went that "a nice, two-for-one Corona at five o'clock happy hour will be ok, and then I'll chill the rest of the night."

I believe, at this point, you're either confused, laughing, or crying. If you are crying, it's all good. I have not had a drink since, and I really don't plan on it anytime soon. I think there are reasons I slipped. The most incredible thing is alcohol is CUNNING, BAFFLING, POWERFUL, and will never stop trying to convince you it's ok. This experiment of mine, one of many, yielded the same results. It is said alcoholism is a progressive disease, and for me, that's 0 to 100, no time flat.

I mentioned earlier I found out in August my Mom had stage 4 lung cancer. When I first found out, I was angry. I was having the time of my life in my own version of Summer Fantasy Triathlon Camp. (Plus, she smoked all those years by choice, didn't she?) I did spend time at the end, but the things I will remember are when she was alive and we would go to the pool with my kids or have dinner together. I am clear with the whole life/death thing. I have spent plenty of time contemplating it.

Originally, I sat down with the intent to write a book to help build my twilight-years job as a triathlon coach. Then it morphed into this addiction memoir. I just felt compelled to tell my story. From the start, I have wanted to reach each one of you. Because I am an addict, I have struggled with ego most of my life, but I have always had equal amounts of fear. I decided to take that fear head-on in this book, as I was reminded at the start of the year by Tony Robins at his UPW event, "Burn the boats, take the island."

Well, I did. Unfortunately, my wife and kids stopped on the beach as I charged ahead. My wife is not as risk tolerant as I am so she was not as committed. This led to my concerns about my own narcissism. I always thought that meant you think of only yourself and want to be the center of attention. I learned a couple of years back, from a man I highly respected as a mentor, how narcissism is so much more than self-centeredness. He got his degree in clinical psychology after he'd retired as an engineer.

Anyway, if you are still practicing your alcoholism, or newly clean, you will have time to ponder some of this later. All indicators are that my behavior in this book could stem from narcissism. Or did? I'm willing to at least sit down at the end of the day and review my behavior and how I may have harmed others. I have honestly believed that my intent and desire, through this process, is to help at least one other person.

This is where I need to keep that ego in check. I can't and couldn't do anything without the help of my Higher Power, who I have no problem identifying as a Christian God. The triathlons, the marathons, food, air—all that stuff provides for a fulfilled life. I'm glad I have a purpose in life and believe I am where I am supposed to be. And right now, the grass looks greener on this side.

About the Author

Shawn was the youngest sibling to his older sister but the middle child during the brief lifetime of his now-deceased baby sister. Shawn did not graduate high school and later earned his GED. College night school filled his schedule during his late '20s and early '30s. Sports have always been a part of Shawn's life, starting with swimming at age 6 until 13 and blossoming into the traditional bat-and-ball sports. A failed attempt at track in high school was followed by distant charity rides on the bike, post-high school, and competitive mogul competitions in his '20s.

Having struggled with addiction problems most of his life, Shawn was finally able to get sober in 2016. Shawn shares his experience, strength, and hope with just about anybody who will listen. His desire to help people achieve their own sobriety is the driving force in his life right now.

As I am putting the final edits to this text, we as a nation are going through something that, in my half century of life, I have never seen before: coronavirus. This makes this book more timely. I had the dream summer; then, in the fall, I spent the end of my mother's life with her, and she passed away on Christmas Eve. Now coronavirus.

As much as this is a book is about overcoming obstacles, that doesn't mean that once you've overcome one that you're done. The next challenge is just on the horizon. The key is to be willing to do your best to get the most personal growth out of each situation and be willing to help others with your experience. The one thing I do know is that since Mexico I have not felt the need to drink; I am very happy going through this crisis sober and lead my family and my church, one day at a time.